T0092597

Atlas of Robotic Prostatectomy

Hubert John • Peter Wiklund
Jorn H. Witt

Editors

Atlas of Robotic Prostatectomy

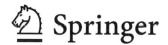 Springer

Editors
Hubert John
Department of Urology
Kantonsspital Winterthur
Winterthur
Switzerland

Peter Wiklund
Department of Urology
Karolinska University Hospital
Stockholm
Sweden

Jorn H. Witt
Department of Urology and Pediatric
Urology-Prostate Center Northwest
St. Antonius-Hospital
Gronau
Germany

ISBN 978-3-540-88407-1   ISBN 978-3-540-88408-8   (eBook)
DOI 10.1007/978-3-540-88408-8
Springer Heidelberg New York Dordrecht London

Library of Congress Control Number: 2012942178

Printed on acid-free paper

Springer is part of Springer Science+Business Media (www.springer.com)

Foreword

It is just 20 years after the first publication of laparoscopic radical prostatectomy by William Schuessler, Ralph Clayman, and Louis Kavoussi in the United States, where the authors stated that this procedure would be too difficult to perform. Only five years later, Richard Gaston, Bertrand Guillonneau, and Guy Vallancien were able to demonstrate the feasibility of the laparoscopic approach mainly because they used an antegrade technique. It took then only three years for Jochen Binder and Claude Abbou to demonstrate the advantages of the da Vinci® system for this procedure. However, it became again necessary to transfer the technique back to the United States to Mani Menon to initiate a surgical revolution which is still taking place in Europe.

Compared to my initial experience as retracting assistant in the early 1980s, when retropubic radical prostatectomy represented a bloody, long-lasting operation done only by the head of the department and his chief-nurse, it is fascinating how video-endoscopic technology has completely transformed the procedure into a bloodless, well-standardized operation where everyone is able to watch every detail of the dissection. Of course, there are many factors that contributed to this success, such as increasing surgical experience, improved knowledge and appreciation of anatomical details, and, last but not least, robotic assistance providing magnification, 3D visualization, and almost unrestricted dexterity in the pelvis.

Therefore, I am sure that it is exactly the right time for this atlas highlighting all important steps of the procedure using state-of-the-art video technology including 3D animations. This will provide a solid basis for the next generation of surgeons who definitively have to learn the robotic technique. Even if some conservative urologists still believe that the open retropubic radical prostatectomy will survive, the train has already left the station....

I congratulate the editors of the atlas for their efforts to focus all the knowledge in superior quality and I am convinced every reader will strongly benefit from it.

Prof. Dr. med. Dr. h.c. Jens Rassweiler
Chairman of Department of Urology
SLK Kliniken Heilbronn
Chairman of EAU-section of Uro-technology (ESUT)

Preface

Radical prostatectomy is the first-line treatment of organ-confined prostate cancer.

The first da Vinci® assisted radical prostatectomy was performed in 2000 based on the combined experiences of conventional laparoscopy and open surgery. Improvement of magnification, three-dimensional imaging, articulated instruments, and precise motor control are still the prime factors that help overcome the potential limitations of conventional laparoscopy. It is then hardly surprising that in the last decade this robotic-assisted technology has expanded its borders well beyond the start-up core of urology and cardiac surgery and found its place with a very broad spectrum of surgeons.

Radical prostatectomy is the most-performed procedure in robotic urology. In the United States, in 2011, about 85% of radical prostatectomies were performed robotically, as experienced open surgeons are able to successfully perform this procedure using this technology, even if lacking laparoscopic experience.

Distinct ablative and reconstructive steps vary considerably in each radical prostatectomy reflecting individual oncologic and functional conditions and underline the complexity of this major surgery. This atlas demonstrates visually rather than through text all the relevant steps of a radical prostatectomy.

The authors have invested great effort and personal experience in showing their individual techniques and we are very grateful to them all for their excellent contributions.

Our special thanks go to our illustrator Stefan Schwyter, Zurich, and video technician Frank Beger, Cologne, who animated graphically the intra-operative moments to an understandable art-form, as well as to Kevin Horton, Winterthur and Mustapha Addali and Jörg Möllers, Gronau, for assisting in the editorial work.

We thank Ms Dörthe Mennecke-Bühler and Ms Meike Stoeck from Springer who helped us to advance the project significantly.

We are especially grateful to our families for their unfaltering support and inexhaustible patience, and we hope that you, dear reader, will enjoy and profit from this atlas of radical prostatectomy.

Winterthur, Switzerland   Hubert John
Stockholm, Sweden   Peter Wiklund
Gronau, Germany   Jorn H. Witt

Contents

Authors and Contributors

Mustapha Addali Department of Urology and Pediatric Urology-Prostate Center Northwest, St. Antonius-Hospital, Gronau, Germany

Thomas E. Ahlering Department of Urology, University of California, Orange, CA, USA

Randy Fagin Intuitive Surgical Inc, Sunnyvale, CA, USA

Rolf Gillitzer Department of Urology, Medical Center Darmstadt, Darmstadt, Germany

Angelika Jansen Department of Anesthesiology, St. Antonius-Hospital, Gronau, Germany

Hubert John Department of Urology, Kantonsspital Winterthur, Winterthur, Switzerland

Apostolos P. Labanaris Department of Urology and Pediatric Urology-Prostate Center Northwest, St. Antonius-Hospital, Gronau, Germany

Günter Lippert Department of Anesthesiology, St. Antonius-Hospital, Gronau, Germany,

Mani Menon Vattikuti Urology Institute Henry Ford Health System, Detroit, MI, USA

Alexander Mottrie Urology Centre, OLV Aalst, Aalst, Belgium

Robert P. Myers Department of Urology, Mayo Clinic, Rochester, MN, USA

Mohan Nathan Intuitive Surgical Inc, Sunnyvale, CA, USA

Vipul R. Patel Florida Hospital, Global Robotics Institute, Celebration, FL, USA

Bernardo Rocco Division of Urology, European Institute of Oncology, Milan, Italy

Charles-Henry Rochat Clinique générale beaulieu, Geneva, Switzerland

Alok Shrivastava Department of Urology, Weston, FL, USA

Stefan Siemer Clinic for Urology and Pediatric Urology, University of Saarland, Homburg/Saar, Germany

Michael Stöckle Clinic for Urology and Pediatric Urology, University of Saarland, Homburg/Saar, Germany

Gerald Tan Weill Cornell Medical Center, Urologic Health Center, New York, NY, USA

Ashutosh K. Tewari Weill Cornell Medical Center, Urologic Health Center, New York, NY, USA

Joachim W. Thüroff Department of Urology, University Medical Center, Mainz, Germany

Peter Wiklund Department of Urology, Karolinska University Hospital, Stockholm, Sweden

Christian Wagner Department of Urology and Pediatric Urology, St. Antonius-Hospital-Prostate Center Northwest, Gronau, Germany

Jorn H. Witt Department of Urology and Pediatric Urology, St. Antonius-Hospital-Prostate Center Northwest, Gronau, Germany

Vahudin Zugor Department of Urology and Pediatric Urology-Prostate Center Northwest, St. Antonius-Hospital, Gronau, Germany

Anatomy: Anatomic Considerations for Efficiency and Precision in Robotic-Assisted Radical Prostatectomy

1

Robert P. Myers

Abbreviations

BPH	Benign prostatic hyperplasia
DF	Denonvilliers' fascia
DVC	Dorsal vein (vascular) complex
FTAP	Fascial tendinous arch of pelvis
LAF	Levator ani fascia
NVB	Neurovascular bundle
PF	Prostatic fascia
PL	Pubovesical/puboprostatic ligament
PSM	Positive surgical margin
RARP	Robotic-assisted radical prostatectomy
SV	Seminal vesicle

Practical success in performing laparoscopic robotic-assisted radical prostatectomy (RARP) depends on the ability of the surgeon to recognize and to preserve anatomic structures contiguous to the prostate that are essential not only for cure of disease but also for excellent functional outcomes.

The three outstanding advantages of laparoscopic RARP are (1) ease of pelvic access without a significant pelvimetry issue (Hong et al. 2009), (2) a relatively dry field due to venous tamponade afforded by carbon dioxide intraperitoneal insufflation, and (3) magnified view in the range of 10–30×. This last advantage brings the surgeon very close to the relevant surgical anatomy, but the admonition of Walsh still holds: "You only see what you are looking for and you only look for what you know" (Walsh 2006).

With a goal of practical application, this review expands on a recent detailed review of surgical anatomy relevant to radical prostatectomy (Walz et al. 2010). Surgical anatomic principles are specifically emphasized for efficiency and precision in dissection in order to avoid a positive surgical margin (PSM), while ultimately achieving urinary control and erectile function once the retropubic space has been accessed using the pubic bone as a landmark.

1.1 Retropubic Space

After port placement and docking of the robot, RARP is begun by taking down distal peritoneum, including transection of the umbilical ligaments, and then developing the retropubic space from the vasa deferentia proximally to the pubic symphysis distally and laterally to the iliac vessels and the parietal endopelvic fascia. Dissection to isolate the prostate and seminal vesicles cannot proceed expeditiously without first removing all retropubic adipose tissue, including loose areolar (cotton candy–like) tissue attached to the visceral fascia covering anterolaterally the bladder and the dorsal vein (vascular) complex (DVC) of the penis. Emerging distally from the fascia, the pubovesical/puboprostatic ligaments (PLs) containing cores of pubovesical muscle attach to the distal third of the pubis (Myers 2002). If these ligaments are partially and proximally transected, the prostate apex drops to facilitate delineation of the anterior prostato-urethral junction, with greatest benefit when there is concomitant benign

H. John, et al. (eds.), *Atlas of Robotic Prostatectomy*,
DOI 10.1007/978-3-540-88408-8_1, © Springer-Verlag Berlin Heidelberg 2013

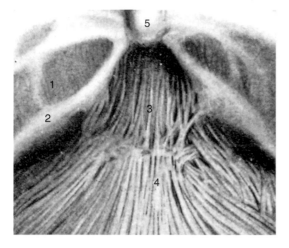

Fig. 1.1 View into retropubic space. *1* Levator ani covered by parietal endopelvic fascia; *2* fascial tendinous arch of pelvis; *3* detrusor apron over underlying prostate with visceral endopelvic fascia removed; *4* longitudinal detrusor muscle of urinary bladder wall; *5* pubic symphysis (From Gil Vernet (1968). Used with permission)

prostatic hyperplasia (BPH). To reapproximate the function of the ligaments to support the urethra distally (Steiner 1994), the ligated DVC can be sutured to the symphysis pubis, a maneuver culminating in some suspension of the underlying urethral stump (Walsh and Partin 2007). However, ultimate impact on urinary continence is not clear. But fixation of the striated sphincter-membranous urethral complex by adjacent subpubic fascia and medial fascia of the levator ani appears to be an important structural mechanism that should be preserved (Burnett and Mostwin 1998).

The surface of visceral endopelvic fascia proximal to the PLs covers longitudinal muscle extension of bladder over prostate, the detrusor apron (Myers 2002), which spreads laterally to each fascial tendinous arch of the pelvis (FTAP) (arcus tendineus fasciae pelvis, *Terminologia Anatomica* [Federative Committee on Anatomical Terminology 1998]) and, in turn, hides underlying DVC and prostate (Fig. 1.1). In most cases (about 90%) (Myers 1991), a superficial vein emerges from the underlying DVC between the PLs to enter retropubic adipose tissue and, in most cases, joins the vesicovenous plexus.

Sometimes the superficial vein emerges to course right or left along the pelvic sidewall.

This then is the initial operative field. The usual full space for RARP working elements extends anteriorly above collapsed bladder to the PLs, laterally to the iliac vessels, deep enough bilaterally to expose the obturator nerves and internal iliac lymph nodes along the internal iliac artery, and, in most cases at the start of the case, proximally to the vasa deferentia descending from each spermatic cord.

1.2 Prostate, BPH, and Pinch Test Variability

Visible impression of the prostate pushing upward against the distal bladder and its anterior detrusor apron becomes increasingly apparent the greater the degree of underlying BPH. BPH contributes directly to the size of the bridge of prostate tissue connecting the halves of the prostate anterior to the urethra, the anterior commissure, the first variable of practical importance to affect the pinch test, which is done by compressing the bladder and its underlying lumen proximal to the prostate with the robotic arms in order to find the optimal point of anterior bladder entry relative to the underlying prostate. Compared with an average prostate with a broader commissure (Fig. 1.2a), the presence of a narrower anterior commissure results in a pinch test showing the bladder lumen to be much closer to the PL takeoff and the prostato-urethral junction (Fig. 1.2b). Conversely, when there is significant protrusion superiorly of BPH, the bladder, like a hood, will encapsulate the prostate. The upwardly protruding BPH (Figs. 1.2c, d) will then make the pinch test less reliable in finding the correct plane of dissection of bladder from prostate without cutting down into the prostate. Furthermore, once the bladder is opened anteriorly, a median lobe of BPH must be recognized when present. Proximity of a median lobe to the interureteric ridge is variable and should be appreciated before incising the

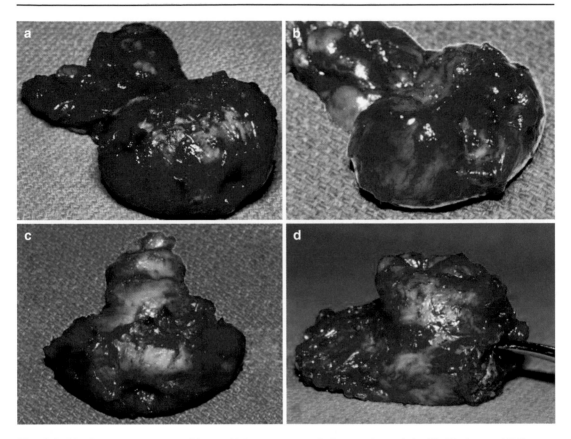

Fig. 1.2 (**a**) Common prostate with toroidal apex. (**b**) Less common prostate with anterior apical notch, posterior lip, and thin anterior commissure. (**c**) Small prostate with benign prostatic hyperplasia (*BPH*) protrusion superiorly toward preexisting bladder lumen. (**d**) Prostate with 90° angulation of urethra at veru such that the anterior surface of prostate consists of circumferential BPH protrusion toward preexisting bladder lumen

posterior bladder wall enroute to the seminal vesicles (SVs).

Also affecting the vesicoprostatic junction is the degree of anterior angulation of the prostatic urethra at the veru, described on average to be 140° (Fig. 1.3b) (McNeal 1972). However, sometimes there is no angle, and at other times the angle may be nearly 90°, a configuration that makes delineation of the vesicoprostatic junction difficult (Fig. 1.2d). The practical point is that the angle affects how BPH projects into the bladder lumen as the prostate elevates the bladder base, including the trigone. If there is no angle and no BPH, the pinch test is very reliable, as opposed to any situation in which there is BPH (Figs. 1.2c, d and 1.3). If bladder entry is made too distal, the anterior prostate may be entered, and if entry is too proximal, the bladder may not reach the urethral stump easily for anastomosis.

1.3   Dorsal Vein (Vascular) Complex

With carbon dioxide pressure, control of the DVC is much simpler than in open surgery, and blood loss is potentially less. Thus, in RARP, control of the DVC, as a result of surgeon preference, may be either immediate or delayed toward the end of the procedure, and at times the DVC may be sectioned without any significant back-bleeding. What is important about the DVC is its variability after emerging proximally from the pubic arch. The safest concept to have in mind is to consider the prostate apex embedded in a nest

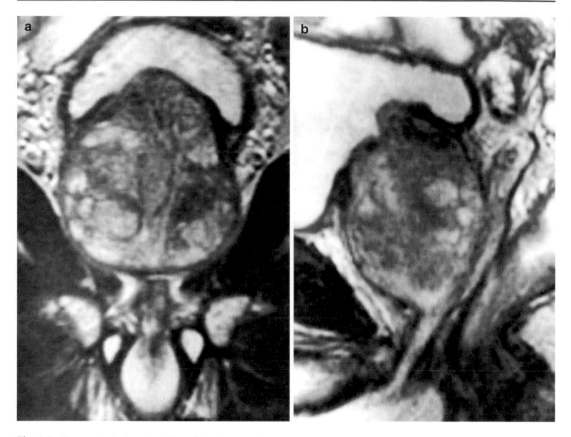

Fig. 1.3 For surgical planning, T2-weighted magnetic resonance coronal (**a**) and sagittal (**b**) images of prostate with benign prostatic hyperplasia protrusion into bladder lumen including median lobe

of veins situated anterior, posterior, and lateral to the apex. These veins then become distributed cephalad into three basic subgroups. The major primary mass of veins and venous sinuses passes anterolaterally on the prostate beneath the detrusor apron, and posterolaterally two minor groups of veins run as elements of the neurovascular bundles (NVBs). As these three groups course cephalad, connections between the posterolateral and anterolateral veins are common. They are readily observed beneath the remnant levator ani fascia (LAF) on the lateral surface of the prostate (see below). Variability is such that the sides of the prostate may be bare of or completely covered with veins. When the lateral surfaces of the prostate are covered by veins, both hemostasis and dissection of the NVB from the posterolateral aspect of the prostate are more complicated.

1.4 Accessory and/or Aberrant Pudendal Arteries

As the retropubic space is cleared of adipose tissue, accessory and/or aberrant pudendal arteries should be recognized and saved whenever possible. Cadaveric study suggests that 70% of men have penile arteries that are both infralevator and supralevator, 15% have exclusively infralevator arteries, and 15% have only supralevator arteries (Droupy et al. 1997). Supralevator pudendal artery origin includes branches from obturator, internal, and external

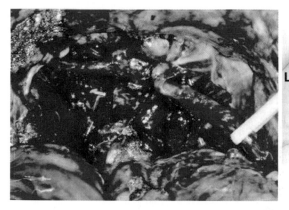
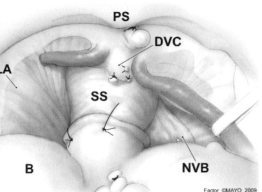

Fig. 1.4 Apical (*left*) and lateral (*right*) supralevator pudendal arteries in relation to striated sphincter and dorsal vein (vascular) complex (*DVC*) after completion of vesicourethral anastomosis. *B* bladder, *LA* levator ani, *NVB* neurovascular bundle, *PS* pubic symphysis, *SS* striated sphincter (Used with permission of Mayo Foundation for Medical Education and Research)

iliac arteries (Walz et al. 2010). These arteries usually course along the side of the bladder if internal iliac in origin, arise often from the obturator artery and run laterally along the pelvic sidewall, or sometimes emerge from the levator ani as apical pudendal arteries (Fig. 1.4) (Mulhall et al. 2008; Walz et al. 2010). Rarely, they derive from a branch of the external iliac artery. These arteries usually enter distally anterior to the DVC and are protected if DVC control is posterior and proximal to the point of pudendal artery entry.

Radical prostatectomy is performed in an age range of men with gradually declining erectile function, particularly after age 60 for various reasons, one of them being atherosclerosis affecting penile blood supply with resultant arterial insufficiency. It is easy to appreciate intraoperatively large supralevator pudendal arteries, but also present are small arteries that accompany each NVB and those associated with the DVC, the latter necessarily transected in the course of any retropubic approach. The combined flow of arterial blood through these small arteries may be critical to erectile function in some men undergoing RARP, and their loss precipitates enough arterial compromise to induce arteriogenic impotence (Mulhall et al. 2008). Preservation of as many supralevator arteries as possible is strongly recommended. The intrafascial dissection described below, which may not be oncologically as safe in some cases, may be more preserving of the fine arterial vasculature and the autonomic nerves that accompany each NVB.

1.5 Vascular Pedicles, NVBs, and Seminal Vesicles

Partially beneath where the DVC more proximally forms a rich plexus of veins at the vesicoprostatic junction (proximal runoff) (Fig. 1.5) (Thomson Walker 1905–06; Beneventi and Noback 1949; Reiner and Walsh 1979), the main vascular pedicle enters the base of the prostate, and the NVBs, very thick at this site, converge with the vessels to form a neurovascular triangle (Takenaka et al. 2006). To preserve the neurovascular triangle with its sympathetic and parasympathetic nerves and numerous ganglia, both the venous plexuses of the DVC runoff and the prostate vascular pedicle must be secured and transected anterior to the main course of the NVBs (Walsh et al. 1983). The correct line of dissection should hug athermally the vesicoprostatic junction and not wander proximally to violate the triangle (Fig. 1.6).

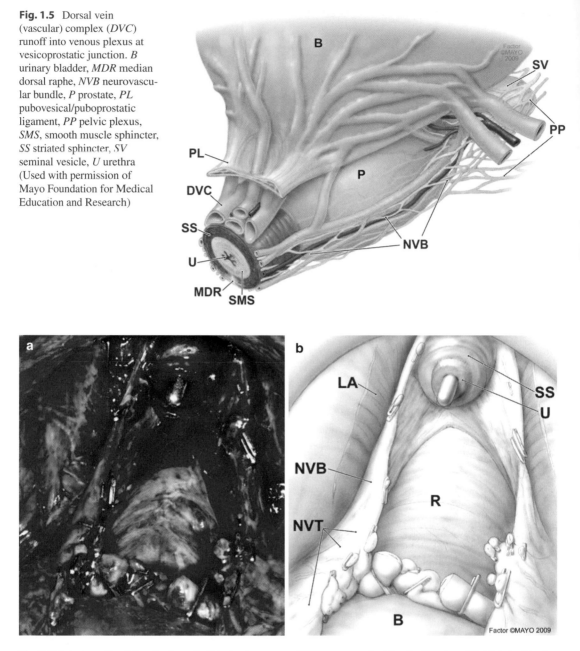

Fig. 1.5 Dorsal vein (vascular) complex (*DVC*) runoff into venous plexus at vesicoprostatic junction. *B* urinary bladder, *MDR* median dorsal raphe, *NVB* neurovascular bundle, *P* prostate, *PL* pubovesical/puboprostatic ligament, *PP* pelvic plexus, *SMS*, smooth muscle sphincter, *SS* striated sphincter, *SV* seminal vesicle, *U* urethra (Used with permission of Mayo Foundation for Medical Education and Research)

Fig. 1.6 Intraoperative (**a**) and schematic (**b**) view: neurovascular bundles (*NVBs*) with neurovascular triangles proximally and high anterior release and posterior decussation distally around urethral stump. *B* bladder, *LA* levator ani, *NVT* neurovascular triangle, *R* rectum, *SS* striated sphincter, *U* urethra with smooth muscle sphincter around protruding tip of 18 Ch (Van Buren sound. Used with permission of Mayo Foundation for Medical Education and Research)

The SVs should always be dissected medially away from the laterally adherent distal portion of the pelvic plexus and subsequent neurovascular tissue (Fig. 1.7). The SVs are tightly bound by nerves not just posterolaterally but also laterally and anterolaterally (Durward 1953; van der Zypen 1988; Lunacek et al. 2005; Walz et al. 2010), and they descend backward and downward in a plane aimed at the S2, S3, and S4 sacral foramina (Fig. 1.8). This plane is different from the coronally

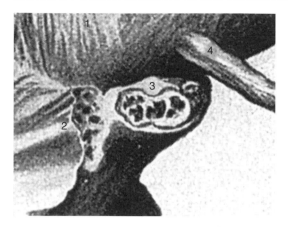

Fig. 1.7 Vascular pedicle, neurovascular bundle, and left seminal vesicle interface. *1* Bladder, *2* neurovascular bundle, *3* left seminal vesicle, *4* ureter (From Gil Vernet (1968). Used with permission)

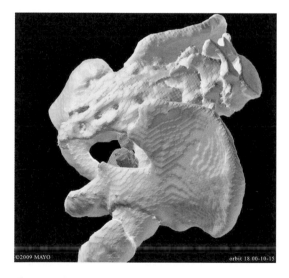

Fig. 1.8 Composite computed tomogram-nuclear magnetic resonance image. Seminal vesicles are directed at S2-4 foramina in plane different from that of prostate (Used with permission of Mayo Foundation for Medical Education and Research)

oriented plane of the prostate as it sits on the rectal surface. A "spray distribution" for nerves of the NVBs has been described occurring just distal to the vascular pedicle (Takenaka et al. 2004), but there is clearly an NVB component adherent to the lateral SV entering the neurovascular triangle, and presumably through numerous ganglia in this region connecting with nerves entering more

distal to the pedicle as a presumptive merging point for sympathetic nerves of hypogastric plexus origin and parasympathetic nerves (nervi erigentes).

Of importance, the actual tips of the SVs are encased in tiny fascial pockets and therefore free from pelvic plexus adherence, which occurs along the lateral surface of the SVs, not at their tips. Saving the tips per se does not translate into preservation of erectile function.

Arterial supply to the SVs is variable. Multiple small arteries to the SVs may enter laterally, at the tips, and medially. Between each SV and vas deferens lies a constant, relatively larger vascular pedicle of arteries and veins supplying both SVs and vasa deferentia.

Distally, the NVBs may decussate or cross-communicate in the midline beneath the posterior prostato-urethral junction (Costello et al. 2004; Takenaka et al. 2006), which bears on Rocco stitch placement posteriorly to anchor the bladder to the rectal serosa (Rocco et al. 2006). Decussation also affects nerve-sparing radical perineal prostatectomy (Weldon et al. 1997) if the decussation has to be disrupted in the midline to find the posterior prostato-urethral junction.

1.6   Denonvilliers' Fascia

The posterior prostate and SVs are covered by a continuous triangular fascia to be entitled herein as the common parlance, eponymic Denonvilliers' fascia (DF), the posterior prostate fascia/seminal vesicles fascia (Walz et al. 2010) or, easier to say, prostatoseminal vesicular fascia (Myers and Villers 2006). The distal tip of this triangular fascia ends in a multilayered terminal plate posterior to the prostato-urethral junction (Stamey 1994). The plate then becomes continuous with the midline, fibrous tissue raphe of the central tendon of the perineum into which the posterior fibers of the striated urethral sphincter insert.

The junction of SVs and prostate posteriorly is the most frequent site of extraprostatic extension of cancer (Jewett et al. 1972). In the interest of oncologic safety, this junction should not be rendered devoid of fascia, meaning that the point of transverse transection of DF in RARP should be performed proximal to the base of the SVs so that there is sufficient fascia on the specimen to cover the vesicoprostatic junction and the posterior surface of the prostate. The correct plane of dissection must be sought carefully. Direct invasion by cancer of this posterior fascia is not common but is of sufficient incidence, especially in cT3 disease, that resection of the prostate should not exclude it as a posterior cover of the underlying peripheral zone capsule (Villers et al. 1993).

Where DF is cut transversely both proximally and distally weighs on the issue of where and how to place sutures for posterior stabilization of the bladder and urethra before vesicourethral anastomosis (Rocco et al. 2006). Parenthetically, although the SVs are covered posteriorly by DF, a true anterior layer of this same fascia on the SVs is a misconception (Secin et al. 2007).

1.7   Prostate, Fascia, and Oncologic Safety

How the prostate should be approached with respect to its surrounding fascias is no small issue with respect to avoiding a PSM but at the same time trying to preserve the NVBs (Stolzenburg et al. 2007). Understanding of the fascia encompassing the prostate is facilitated by appreciating that there are basically two primary layers, an outer LAF and an inner visceral, frequently multilayered, prostatic fascia (PF) with nerves, arteries, and veins sandwiched in between the two layers (Walz et al. 2010). In essentially half of cases (52%), the layers are separated, and in the remaining half (48%), there is an element of fusion of outer and inner layers (Kiyoshima et al. 2004). Within these two layers, autonomic nerves, some destined for the corpora cavernosa, are variably distributed along the lateral and posterolateral prostate, and the vessels provide scaffolding to form the bundles and a visual landmark for the course of the nerves with respect to NVB preservation (Walsh et al. 1983). In addition, Kiyoshima et al. (2004) found a discrete NVB at the posterolateral prostate in only 52% of cases, whereas in the other 48% the nerves were more

evenly distributed over the lateral surfaces of the prostate. This latter configuration provided justification for the Veil of Aphrodite dissection by Kaul et al. (2005) and the curtain dissection by Lunacek et al. (2005).

Eichelberg et al. (2007) counted the nerves per prostate half and found 21–28% of nerves on the anterior half. With computerized planimetry, Ganzer et al. (2008) found nerve surface area to be highest posterolaterally, but with a range of 40% anterolaterally to 46% posteriorly. Kaiho et al. (2009) performed intraoperative electrophysiologic stimulation along the lateral surface of the mid-prostate at 1, 2, 3, 4, and 5 o'clock with the finding of increasing amplitude of corpus spongiosum tumescence from 1 to 5 o'clock as monitored by an intraurethral pressure sensor. High anterior release of the LAF is associated with better erectile function outcomes (Nielsen et al. 2008). The more fascia that is preserved, the better seems to be the outcome (van der Poel and de Blok 2009). All these studies support high anterior release of the LAF, as illustrated for open surgery by Montorsi et al. (2005).

From a surgical standpoint, in order to pinpoint the precise anterior edge of the underlying NVB, the distribution of veins on the mid-lateral surface of the prostate beneath the LAF provides a guide. Veins associated with the NVB usually run, beyond the vascular pedicle, on the lateral and posterolateral prostate parallel to the rectum and then swing up distally at the prostate apex to flank the urethral stump as far as the 11- and 1-o'clock positions (Fig. 1.6).

In RARP, initially it is possible to begin to free the prostate by incising the endopelvic fascia either lateral or medial to the FTAP. An incision lateral to the FTAP, the common approach of open surgery, provides a plane of dissection that results in the entire lateral surface of the prostate being covered initially by LAF. An incision medial to the FTAP allows entry medial to the LAF and additionally medial to PF covering prostate capsule, which is the outer smooth muscle layer of fibromuscular stroma, when present. By definition, this medial approach becomes intrafascial relative to the NVB and leaves the FTAP in situ and intact as an anchor point for continuous suture approximation of the bladder for anterior stabilization of the bladder after completion of the RARP anastomosis (Tewari et al. 2007).

The potential trouble with a fundamentally intrafascial approach is that surgeons have no clue as they dissect with respect to fascia-capsule variability (Walz et al. 2010), which can change at any moment during fascial mobilization. If great care is not exercised, an onion-skinning effect affecting multilayered, periprostatic fascia and capsule is possible from the fine dissection capability of RARP, and this may cause confusion and thus make it necessary to try a different line of dissection in the quest to avoid a PSM.

Of note, prostate capsule may be absent in places bringing glands in direct contact with periprostatic tissue (Epstein 2001). Should cancer be present at one of these points and an intrafascial approach used, a PSM is certain if cancer is at that margin. Of further complexity is the fact that prostate capsule and contiguous PF may interdigitate and thus make it impossible to develop an intrafascial plane without ending up in the prostate (inadvertent prostate incision or capsulotomy). The range of variation from capsule-no PF to PF-no capsule with variable combinations will confound the best of surgeons (Walz et al. 2010). And it may just be a matter of luck if a PSM is avoided with an intrafascial dissection if cases are not chosen carefully based on preoperative clinical findings. The posterolateral margin of dissection is particularly treacherous when there is only a single layer of PF between prostate and NVB (Kourambas et al. 1998). The interfascial dissection therefore is ultimately the safest in terms of preventing PSMs, and it is furthermore a consideration when NVBs are stuck to the prostate by inflammatory adherence.

With respect to dissection and degrees of preservation of periprostatic fascia and NVB, four approaches are now described and illustrated (Fig. 1.9). The first approach is to be completely intrafascial with respect to the entire prostate and SVs. This dissection is the least oncologically safe, the most nerve- and vessel-preserving, and a prominent feature of the Veil or curtain dissections (Kaul et al. 2005; Lunacek et al. 2005; Walz et al. 2010).

The second approach to prostate removal is modified intrafascial and NVB-sparing but with the exception that DF is preserved and covers the majority of the posterior surface of the final prostate specimen. This is an important consideration in men with larger tumors for which DF invasion by cancer is a significant risk (Villers et al. 1993).

During this approach, there is a choice of leaving the anteromedial surface of the NVB uncovered or covered by fascia. In order to understand this best, consider that DF, after midline fusion in 97% of cases (Kiyoshima et al. 2004), splits laterally into just two layers, one anterior and one posterior with respect to the NVB, with the anterior layer as PF covering and sharing simultaneously the posterolateral prostate and anteromedial surface of the adjacent NVB. If dissection allows this shared layer to stay with the adjacent anteromedial surface of the NVB, the adjacent posterolateral prostate capsule will be denuded of fascia. The result is potentially more nerve-preserving but less oncologically safe. Because this dissection passes anterior to both anterior and posterior layers of DF, the dissection is termed *intrafascial* with respect to the NVB (Myers and Villers 2006).

Alternatively, in a third approach, this shared layer of PF can be left to cover the posterolateral prostate leaving the NVB denuded of fascia. The idea is to dissect so that the entire prostate will be covered by PF. This dissection necessarily passes between the anterior and posterior layers of DF described above and is termed *interfascial*. The anteromedial surface of the NVB will be visibly devoid of fascia. This approach may be less nerve-preserving and less preserving of the very fine arterial vasculature of the NVB, but it is particularly applicable in palpable cT2 disease in order to prevent a PSM. The most important and largest pro-erectile nerves (nervi erigentes) can be preserved with the interfascial approach if they are not interrupted for some reason at the line of dissection. Parenthetically, the NVB is usually tethered at the prostato-urethral angle by a vessel, a special point of release necessary for successful preservation (Walsh and Partin 2007).

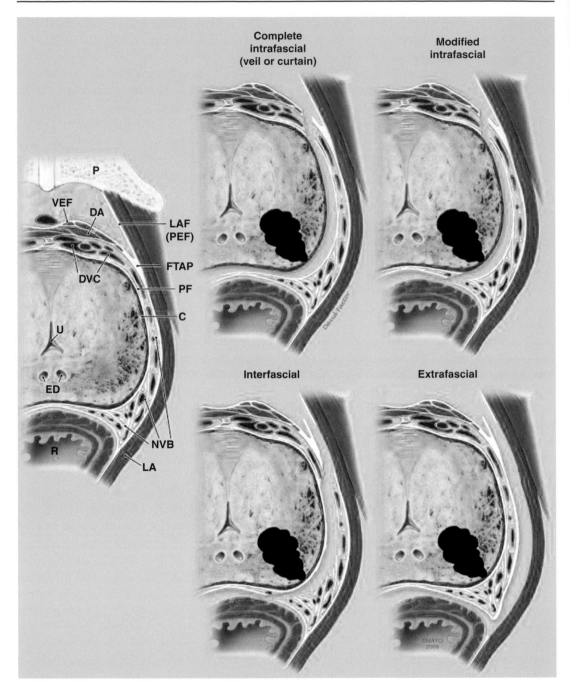

Fig. 1.9 Four different fascial dissections with respect to neurovascular bundle (*NVB*), prostatic fascia (*PF*), and levator ani fascia (*LAF*). *C* capsule, *DA* detrusor apron, *DVC* dorsal vein (vascular) complex, *ED* ejaculatory ducts, *FTAP* fascial tendinous arch of pelvis, *LA* levator ani, *LAF* (*PEF*) levator ani fascia (parietal endopelvic fascia), *P* prostate, *R* rectum, *U* urethra, *VEF* visceral endopelvic fascia (Used with permission of Mayo Foundation for Medical Education and Research)

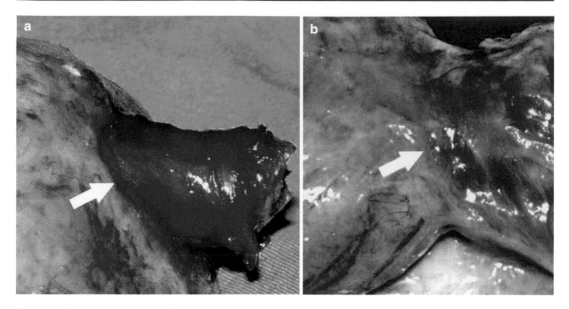

Fig. 1.10 Clear (**a**) and unclear (**b**) delineation of prostate-striated sphincter interface (*arrows*)

The fourth approach is the wide, non-nerve-sparing resection for extensive cT2 and cT3 disease. The posterior layer of DF passes posterior to the NVB and fuses laterally with LAF, which covers the lateral surface of the NVB. This configuration thereby creates a triangle of fascia investing the NVB. This fourth type of dissection is carried external to all layers of fascia investing the NVB and is therefore termed *extrafascial*, the most oncologically safe in terms of not obtaining a PSM.

1.8   Prostate Apex

Dissection at the prostate apex is confounded by uncertain delineation of the prostate-striated sphincter interface in many cases (Fig. 1.10) and further by variation in the shape of the prostate apex and overlap of the striated sphincter and underlying membranous urethra by distal growth of the prostate. At times the interface is clear, and usually more so when there is BPH. If overlap, both posterior and anterior, is not recognized and accounted for in dissection, there is a risk of both a PSM and insufficient residual urethral length for continence (Fig. 1.11).

Patients with overlap of their sphincter by prostate, as shown by preoperative T2-weighted magnetic resonance imaging, have been shown to have a significantly increased incidence of urinary incontinence at 3 months after surgery (Lee et al. 2006).

The average prostate is surgically easy to dissect with a clear point of urethral transection at the apex (Fig. 1.2a). Small prostates with anterior apical notches and posterior lips overlapping the urethral stump posteriorly or from underneath have NVBs situated more lateral on the prostate as they approach the prostato-urethral junction (Figs. 1.2b and 1.11a). The posterior lip situation is in contrast to significant BPH that overlaps the prostato-urethral junction anteriorly and is associated with a relatively massive anterior commissure. In such cases, the NVBs can be expected to be more posterolateral with respect to the urethral stump (Figs. 1.2d and 1.11b).

Any degree of overlap affects surgical technique in preserving the full functional length of the urethral stump, the mission being to exercise correct judgment in deciding where to divide the urethra anteriorly and then posteriorly. From a practical standpoint, in order to

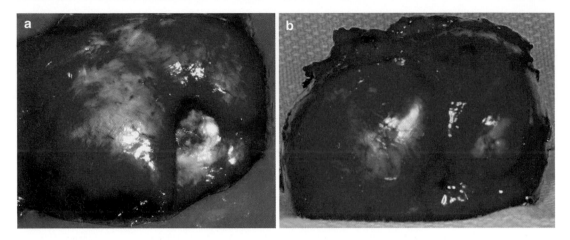

Fig. 1.11 (**a**) Apex with typical anterior apical notch and posterior lip overlap of preexisting urethral stump. (**b**) Apex with anterior benign prostatic hyperplasia overlap of preexisting urethral stump

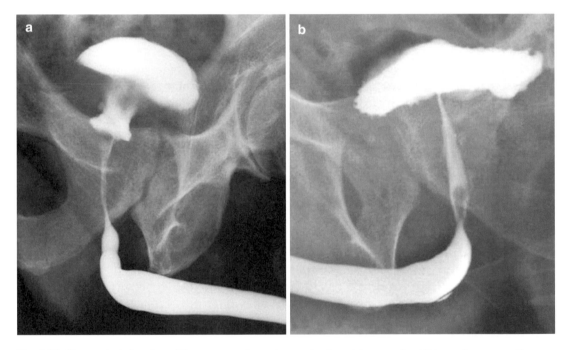

Fig. 1.12 For surgical planning, oblique retrograde urethrography: long (**a**) versus short (**b**) membranous urethras

avoid a wrong move, the nature of the prostate-sphincter interface with respect to possible overlap could be investigated preoperatively with T2-weighted magnetic resonance imaging in both coronal and sagittal planes (Fig. 1.3), and membranous urethral length could be determined simply by retrograde urethrography in oblique view (Fig. 1.12).

1.9 Striated Urethral Sphincter and Membranous Urethra

The usual antegrade dissection of RARP must protect the urethral stump in order to optimize the quickest return of urinary control, the surgeon knowing full well that a patient's life may be ruined if he is rendered incontinent of urine. The urethral stump is a cylindrical to conical-shaped structure of variable length that extends from the prostate apex to the corpus spongiosum (bulb) (Myers et al. 1998; Walz et al. 2010).

As measured by preoperative magnetic resonance imaging, it appears necessary to preserve a minimum length of 1.4 cm in the urethral stump for satisfactory continence (Coakley et al. 2002; Paparel et al. 2009). For patients with less than 1.4 cm, it has been shown to be helpful in improving urinary continence by combining both posterior, by the Rocco stitch, and anterior stabilization, by suturing anterior bladder wall to the FTAP, after vesicourethral anastomosis (Nguyen et al. 2008).

The urethral stump components that need protection are what Turner Warwick called the *distal sphincter mechanism* (1983). In the urethral stump (*Terminologia Anatomica*'s *intermediate urethra* [Federative Committee on Anatomical Terminology 1998]), the components consist of the outer external striated urethral sphincter (rhabdosphincter), the inner smooth muscle-elastic tissue of the membranous urethra (lissosphincter), and the delicate papillary infoldings of the mucosa that create a mucosal seal when the urethra is collapsed. Blood and nerve supply are naturally important. Of secondary importance are the ancillary puboperineales (also known as pubourethralis, levator urethrae) (Myers et al. 2000), the thickened bands of levator ani that form the anterior levator (Ayoub 1979) or urogenital (Oelrich 1980) hiatus. They should not be disturbed when the PLs are partially incised because there may be autonomic nerves passing through levator muscle to become cavernous nerve in destination (Müller 1836). Furthermore, the ability to perform Kegel exercises and stop the urinary stream quickly will be compromised.

Optimal urethral transection for urinary continence is based on the following principles: (1) preservation of the full length of the striated sphincter with a realization that its length is variable and may be no more than a centimeter in extreme cases (Fig. 1.12b); (2) anterior transection of the membranous urethra 2–3 mm proximal to the observed beginning or superior

end of the striated sphincter; and (3) posterior transection of the membranous urethra just distal to the veru with the same limitation as utilized and respected in transurethral resection of the prostate. Final release of the prostate from the urethral stump involves transection of the terminal plate of DF, not rectourethralis, which is more distal and centers on the bulbourethral glands. Transection of the urethra more distally leaving 2–3 mm of striated sphincter and underlying membranous urethra attached to the prostate apex is to be frowned on because such strategy to avoid a PSM may leave the patient with insufficient residual urethral length to be continent. Unrecognized prostate-sphincter overlap will only compound.

The striated sphincter is typically thickest anterolaterally and becomes thinner posterolaterally, where it typically inserts into a midline raphe (Fig. 1.13a). The striated sphincter should not be viewed as having uniform circumferential thickness. The 6-o'clock position is the weakest site to hold a suture securely and the most common site of a urinary leak; thus, with forethought, suture placement in the RARP technique should bridge, but close, the 6-o'clock position.

The urethral stump has supporting lateral fascia, including the variable appearance of lateral fascial bands (Walsh's pillars [Walsh 1986]) into which the anterior layer (as opposed to the circumferential layer) of the striated sphincter inserts (Magera et al. 2008). Protecting peri-urethral fascia will help to protect urethral stump integrity.

Undue stretching of the elastic tissue of the membranous urethra should be avoided because it may delay return of urinary control. Trauma from grooved sounds or other devices may disrupt and denude the mucosal seal (Figs. 1.13b, c).

The nerve supply to the urethral stump should be protected and emanates from both infralevator and supralevator pathways (Hollabaugh et al. 1997). Stimulation of the NVBs intraoperatively produces urethral stump contraction (Nelson et al. 2003). Even though it is not necessary to preserve the NVBs for patients to be continent, urinary control has been shown to be significantly improved in patients undergoing NVB preservation (Burkhard et al. 2006).

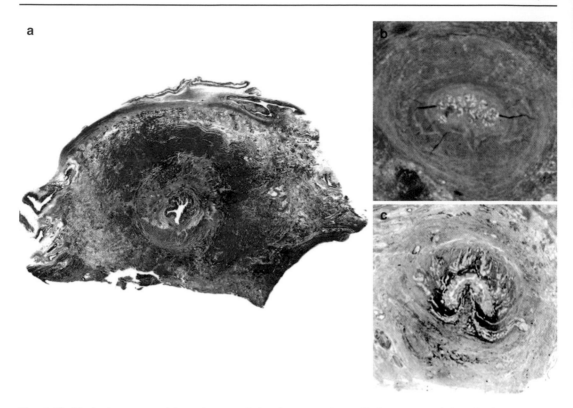

Fig. 1.13 Urethral stump, axial section. (**a**) Striated sphincter (*red*) around membranous urethra with circumferential smooth muscle (Masson trichrome). (**b**) Urethral mucosal "seal" from mucosal invaginations (Masson trichrome). (**c**) Significant elastic tissue (*black*) within membranous urethra (elastic tissue stain)

References

Ayoub SF (1979) The anterior fibres of the levator ani muscle in man. J Anat 128:571–580

Beneventi FA, Noback GJ (1949) Distribution of the blood vessels of the prostate gland and urinary bladder: application to retropubic prostatectomy. J Urol 62:663–671

Burkhard FC, Kessler TM, Fleischmann A et al (2006) Nerve sparing open radical retropubic prostatectomy: does it have an impact on urinary continence? J Urol 176:189–195

Burnett AL, Mostwin JL (1998) In situ anatomical study of the male urethral sphincteric complex: relevance to continence preservation following major pelvic surgery. J Urol 160:1301–1306

Coakley FV, Eberhardt S, Kattan MW et al (2002) Urinary continence after radical retropubic prostatectomy: relationship with membranous urethral length on preoperative endorectal magnetic resonance imaging. J Urol 168:1032–1035

Costello AJ, Brooks M, Cole OJ (2004) Anatomical studies of the neurovascular bundle and cavernosal nerves. BJU Int 94:1071–1076

Droupy S, Benoit G, Giuliano F et al (1997) Penile arteries in humans: origin, distribution, variations. Surg Radiol Anat 19:161–167

Durward A (1953) Abdomino-pelvic plexuses in peripheral nervous system. In: Brash JC (ed) Cunningham's anatomy, 9th edn. Oxford University Press, London

Eichelberg C, Erbersdobler A, Michl U et al (2007) Nerve distribution along the prostatic capsule. Eur Urol 51:105–110

Epstein JI (2001) Pathologic assessment of the surgical specimen. Urol Clin North Am 28:567–594

Federative Committee on Anatomical Terminology (1998) Terminologia anatomica: international anatomical terminology. Thieme, Stuttgart

Ganzer R, Blana A, Gaumann A et al (2008) Topographical anatomy of periprostatic and capsular nerves: quantification and computerised planimetry. Eur Urol 54:353–360

Gil Vernet S (1968) Morphology and function of vesico-prostato-urethral musculature. Canova, Treviso

Hollabaugh RS Jr, Dmochowski RR, Steiner MS (1997) Neuroanatomy of the male rhabdosphincter. Urology 49:426–434

Hong SK, Lee ST, Kim SS et al (2009) Effect of bony pelvic dimensions measured by preoperative magnetic resonance imaging on performing robot-assisted laparoscopic prostatectomy. BJU Int 104:664–668

Jewett HJ, Eggleston JC, Yawn DH (1972) Radical prostatectomy in the management of carcinoma of the prostate: probable causes of some therapeutic failures. J Urol 107:1034–1040

Kaiho Y, Nakagawa H, Saito H et al (2009) Nerves at the ventral prostatic capsule contribute to erectile function: initial electrophysiological assessment in humans. Eur Urol 55:148–155

Kaul S, Bhandari A, Hemal A et al (2005) Robotic radical prostatectomy with preservation of the prostatic fascia: a feasibility study. Urology 66:1261–1265

Kiyoshima K, Yokomizo A, Yoshida T et al (2004) Anatomical features of periprostatic tissue and its surroundings: a histological analysis of 79 radical retropubic prostatectomy specimens. Jpn J Clin Oncol 34:463–468

Kourambas J, Angus DG, Hosking P et al (1998) A histological study of Denonvilliers' fascia and its relationship to the neurovascular bundle. Br J Urol 82:408–410

Lee SE, Byun SS, Lee HJ et al (2006) Impact of variations in prostatic apex shape on early recovery of urinary continence after radical retropubic prostatectomy. Urology 68:137–141

Lunacek A, Schwentner C, Fritsch H et al (2005) Anatomical radical retropubic prostatectomy: 'curtain dissection' of the neurovascular bundle. BJU Int 95:1226–1231

Magera JS Jr, Inman BA, Slezak JM et al (2008) Increased optical magnification from 2.5× to 4.3× with technical modification lowers the positive margin rate in open radical retropubic prostatectomy. J Urol 179:130–135

McNeal JE (1972) The prostate and prostatic urethra: a morphologic synthesis. J Urol 107:1008–1016

Montorsi F, Salonia A, Suardi N et al (2005) Improving the preservation of the urethral sphincter and neurovascular bundles during open radical retropubic prostatectomy. Eur Urol 48:938–945

Mulhall JP, Secin FP, Guillonneau B (2008) Artery sparing radical prostatectomy: myth or reality? J Urol 179:827–831

Müller J (1836) Über die organischen Nerven der erectilen männlichen Geschlectsorgane des Menschen und der Säugethiere [Concerning the autonomic nerves of the male erectile genital organs of man and mammals]. German. F. Dümmler, Berlin

Myers RP (1991) Anatomical variation of the superficial preprostatic veins with respect to radical retropubic prostatectomy. J Urol 145:992–993

Myers RP (2002) Detrusor apron, associated vascular plexus, and avascular plane: relevance to radical retropubic prostatectomy: anatomic and surgical commentary. Urology 59:472–479

Myers RP, Villers A (2006) Anatomic considerations in radical prostatectomy. In: Kirby RS, Partin AW, Feneley M et al (eds) Prostate cancer: principles and practice. Taylor & Francis, London

Myers RP, Cahill DR, Devine RM et al (1998) Anatomy of radical prostatectomy as defined by magnetic resonance imaging. J Urol 159:2148–2158

Myers RP, Cahill DR, Kay PA et al (2000) Puboperineales: muscular boundaries of the male urogenital hiatus in 3D from magnetic resonance imaging. J Urol 164:1412–1415

Nelson CP, Montie JE, McGuire EJ et al (2003) Intraoperative nerve stimulation with measurement of urethral sphincter pressure changes during radical retropubic prostatectomy: a feasibility study. J Urol 169:2225–2228

Nguyen L, Jhaveri J, Tewari A (2008) Surgical technique to overcome anatomical shortcoming: balancing postprostatectomy continence outcomes of urethral sphincter lengths on preoperative magnetic resonance imaging. J Urol 179:1907–1911

Nielsen ME, Schaeffer EM, Marschke P et al (2008) High anterior release of the levator fascia improves sexual function following open radical retropubic prostatectomy. J Urol 180:2557–2564

Oelrich TM (1980) The urethral sphincter muscle in the male. Am J Anat 158:229–246

Paparel P, Akin O, Sandhu JS et al (2009) Recovery of urinary continence after radical prostatectomy: association with urethral length and urethral fibrosis measured by preoperative and postoperative endorectal magnetic resonance imaging. Eur Urol 55:629–637

Reiner WG, Walsh PC (1979) An anatomical approach to the surgical management of the dorsal vein and Santorini's plexus during radical retropubic surgery. J Urol 121:198–200

Rocco F, Carmignani L, Acquati P et al (2006) Restoration of posterior aspect of rhabdosphincter shortens continence time after radical retropubic prostatectomy. J Urol 175:2201–2206

Secin FP, Karanikolas N, Gopalan A et al (2007) The anterior layer of Denonvilliers' fascia: a common misconception in the laparoscopic prostatectomy literature. J Urol 177:521–525

Stamey TA (1994) Techniques for avoiding positive surgical margins during radical prostatectomy. Atlas Urol Clin North Am 2:37–51

Steiner MS (1994) The puboprostatic ligament and the male urethral suspensory mechanism: an anatomic study. Urology 44:530–534

Stolzenburg JU, Schwalenberg T, Horn LC et al (2007) Anatomical landmarks of radical prostatecomy. Eur Urol 51:629–639

Takenaka A, Murakami G, Soga H et al (2004) Anatomical analysis of the neurovascular bundle supplying penile cavernous tissue to ensure a reliable nerve graft after radical prostatectomy. J Urol 172:1032–1035

Takenaka A, Leung RA, Fujisawa M et al (2006) Anatomy of autonomic nerve component in the male pelvis: the new concept from a perspective for robotic nerve sparing radical prostatectomy. World J Urol 24:136–143

Tewari AK, Bigelow K, Rao S et al (2007) Anatomic restoration technique of continence mechanism and preservation of puboprostatic collar: a novel modification to achieve early urinary continence in men undergoing robotic prostatectomy. Urology 69:726–731

Thomson Walker JW (1905–06) On the surgical anatomy of the prostate. J Anat Physiol 40:189–209

Turner Warwick R (1983) The sphincter mechanisms: their relation to prostatic enlargement and its treatment. In: Hinman F Jr (ed) Benign prostatic hypertrophy. Springer, New York

van der Poel HG, de Blok W (2009) Role of extent of fascia preservation and erectile function after robot-assisted laparoscopic prostatectomy. Urology 73:816–821

van der Zypen EM (1988) Composition and topographic anatomy of the inferior hypogastric plexus (pelvic plexus). SANDORAMA III–IV:24–32

Villers A, McNeal JE, Freiha FS et al (1993) Invasion of Denonvilliers' fascia in radical prostatectomy specimens. J Urol 149:793–798

Walsh PC (1986) Urologic surgery: radical retropubic prostatectomy: an anatomic approach with preservation of sexual function. Bristol Laboratories, Syracuse

Walsh PC (2006) Course 25 IC-radial retropubic prostatectomy. Annual urological association meeting, Atlanta, 2006

Walsh PC, Partin AW (2007) Anatomic radical retropubic prostatectomy. In: Wein AJ, Kavoussi LR, Novick AC et al (eds) Campbell-Walsh urology, 9th edn. Saunders/Elsevier, Philadelphia

Walsh PC, Lepor H, Eggleston JC (1983) Radical prostatectomy with preservation of sexual function: anatomical and pathological considerations. Prostate 4:473–485

Walz J, Burnett AL, Costello AJ et al (2010) A critical analysis of the current knowledge of surgical anatomy related to optimization of cancer control and preservation of continence and erection in candidates for radical prostatectomy. Eur Urol 57:179–192

Weldon VE, Tavel FR, Neuwirth H (1997) Continence, potency and morbidity after radical perineal prostatectomy. J Urol 158:1470–1475

Anesthesiology: Anaesthesiological Aspects in the Context of Robot-Assisted Radical Prostatectomy

2

Angelika Jansen and Günter Lippert

2.1   Introduction

Time and again the use of innovative surgical techniques confronts anaesthetists with the task of selecting the most suitable type of anaesthesia for the respective procedure, adapting it to the new requirements and ensuring dependable perioperative patient care by means of a patient-oriented, continuous improvement process. The aim of this chapter is to give a presentation – from practitioners for practitioners – of the standardised anaesthetic procedure that was developed at our hospital and has proven successful in over 1,500 operations, as well as its special features in connection with use of the Da Vinci.

2.2   Before the Operation

As before every operation, a premedication talk is held with the aim of exchanging information. The anaesthetist gets an impression of the current state of health of the patient during this talk, and on the basis of the medical history and the physical examination. At the same time, he informs the patient about the planned anaesthetic procedure in the form of balanced general anaesthesia. An ECG and a laboratory check are performed as standard for further diagnosis. Since our experience shows that a need for intraoperative blood transfusion is not to be expected, there

is no need for corresponding preparatory measures. If a particular cardiac risk is suspected as a result of the premedication talk, further examinations are performed by the in-house cardiologist. The operation should be deferred if this examination reveals therapeutic consequences that could contribute to reducing the cardiac risk. In the event of manifest organ failures that can no longer be improved and substantially impair the patient's stress tolerance (>ASA III), consideration should be given to performing a different therapeutic procedure (e.g. brachytherapy or EBRT). Similarly, obesity that is of a truncal nature, and thus cannot be determined solely on the basis of the BMI, can make the procedure impossible: partly for ventilation-related, i.e. anaesthesiological reasons and partly for positioning and instrument-related, i.e. surgical, reasons.

For preoperative anxiolysis and sedation, the patient is routinely given a benzodiazepine (dipotassium clorazepate [Tranxilium®] 20–30 mg p.o.) on the previous evening and on the day of the operation. The perioperative pain concept commences preoperatively with a COX-2 inhibitor (etoricoxib [Arcoxia®] 1–1.5 mg/kg BW p.o.). Preoperative prophylaxis of postoperative nausea and vomiting (PONV) is performed in corresponding cases by means of the H1 receptor antagonist dimenhydrate 50 mg p.o. and is intraoperatively supplemented by dexamethasone [Fortecortin®] 4 mg i.v. in individual cases.

H. John, et al. (eds.), *Atlas of Robotic Prostatectomy*,
DOI 10.1007/978-3-540-88408-8_2, © Springer-Verlag Berlin Heidelberg 2013

2.3   Operation

2.3.1   Preparation of Anaesthesia

On the day of the operation, the patient is greeted by the anaesthesia nurse and the anaesthetist, the check of his identity and his findings being documented in a special time-out record. After positioning the patient on the operating table equipped with a vacuum mattress, further preparation is performed in the ante-room of the operating theatre.

In addition to the 3-lead ECG, and owing to the apposition of both arms and the 30° Trendelenburg position, the standard provides for a "bilateral procedure": establishment of peripheral venous accesses (17G/18G) on the back of both hands or on both forearms, application of pulse oximetry sensors to the middle finger of both hands, wrapping of both arms in cotton wool to protect against postural damage application of sphygmomanometer cuffs to both upper arms. The two crystalloid infusions (à 500 ml Sterofundin®) connected to the peripheral venous accesses are stopped. Both the risk of a vesicourethral anastomotic leak and the possibility of intraoperative development of cerebral or pulmonary oedema owing to the extreme head-down position are minimised by a restrictive fluid supply.

Only in cases of cardiac risk is the standard extended to include a 5-lead ECG for ST-segment analysis and invasive blood pressure measurement (left-side A. radialis), as well as an external pacemaker and central venous catheter, where appropriate.

Every patient receives a cephalosporin [Cefuroxim® 1.5 g] i.v. as a single-shot antibiotic, alternatively being given ciprofloxacin [Ciprobay® 500 mg], for example, in case of intolerance.

2.3.2   Induction of Anaesthesia

Following connection of the monitoring equipment, anaesthesia is induced in the operating theatre. Norepinephrine is administered by means of a Perfusor syringe pump [Arterenol® 0.02 mg/ml

at 0.1–25 ml/h] to stabilise the haemodynamics. As standard, induction is performed i.v. with Sufenta® 15 μg, propofol 2–2.5 mg/kg BW and rocuronium 0.5 mg/kg BW. Oral intubation is followed by minimal flow ventilation, sevoflurane or desflurane being added. A stomach tube is inserted orally for the duration of the operation to drain the gastric juice. Special protective glasses that fit tightly on all sides are put on to additionally protect the patient's eyes against the possibility of position-induced penetration of fluids, such as blood or gastric juice, during the operation, and simultaneously to prevent drying of the eyes in the event of incomplete lid closure (see Fig. 2.1). A gauze compress inserted into the mouth helps avoid damage to the lips and tongue as a result of exposure to uncontrolled pressure. A nasal temperature sensor permits monitoring of the body temperature, external heat being supplied by means of a thermal blanket. Only then does the team position the patient on the operating table: after bending the legs to the side, both arms are positioned closely against the body and fixed by evacuating the appropriately adjusted vacuum mattress, the head also being fixed on the pillow in this way. The patency of the two infusion systems is subsequently checked once more, after which the systems are stopped again (see Fig. 2.2 and 2.3).

2.3.3   Special Features of Anaesthesia Management

Use of the da Vinci robot for prostatectomy results in a number of special features as regards anaesthesia management.

As already described, the close positioning of the arms against the body can, on the one hand, cause postural damage, meaning that not only gel cushions are important, but also careful padding of the arms. On the other hand, an intraoperative failure of blood pressure measurement, pulse oximetry or the infusion system can lead to the disruption of anaesthesia management and/or interruption of the operation, meaning that prophylactic connection to both arms increases safety.

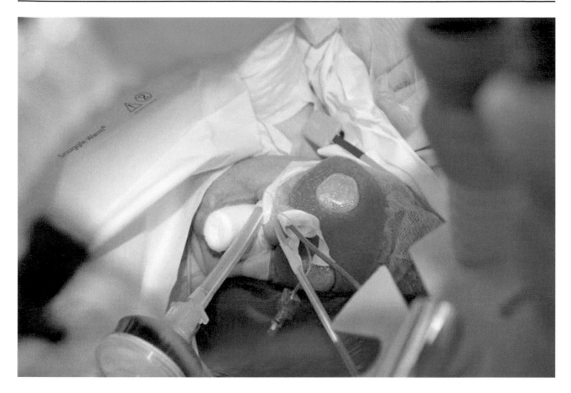

Fig. 2.1   Special protective glasses protect the patient's eyes

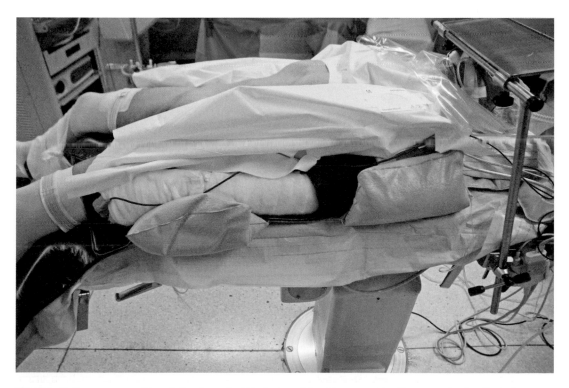

Fig. 2.2   Both arms are positioned closely against the body and fixed by evacuating the appropriately adjusted vacuum mattress

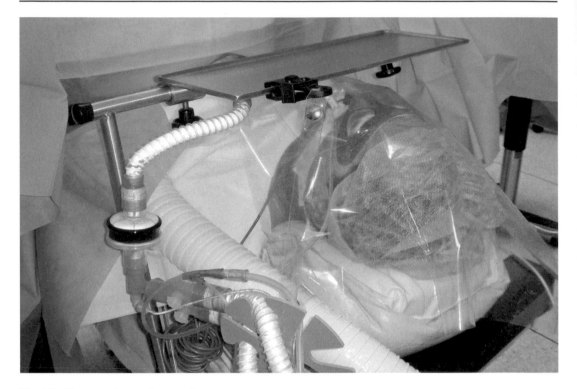

Fig. 2.3 The operation can be started

The operation is performed in a 30° Trendelenburg position (see Fig. 2.4). In combination with creation of the capnoperitoneum, this can from our point of view lead to more or less severe impairment of the haemodynamics, depending on the cardiac stress tolerance of the patient. In their paper, Falabella et al. demonstrated an increase in the mean arterial pressure and the systemic vascular resistance, induced by the head-down position and the capnoperitoneum, along with a simultaneous reduction in the diameter of the aorta (Falabella et al. 2007). According to Meininger et al., the haemodynamic effects of a capnoperitoneum are determined by the level of the intraabdominal pressure, the degree of existing cardiocirculatory and pulmonary diseases, the patient's volume status, the effects of the capnoperitoneum on the acid–base balance and, ultimately, also by the positioning measures required for the operation. Following differential diagnostic exclusion of a gas embolism, the possible occurrence of cardiac arrhythmia when creating

the capnoperitoneum can, according to Meininger et al., be explained by the vagal stimulation caused by the distension of the peritoneum (Meininger and Byhahn 2008). In our own patients, we quite often observe bradycardia with heart rates of less than 40 bpm, which is limited either spontaneously or by giving atropine. However, substantial circulatory reactions with significant drops in blood pressure also occur, these being treated solely by means of norepinephrine, without administering additional volume. A switch to adrenaline [Suprarenin®] has so far only been necessary in a few isolated cases, and premature discontinuation of the operation after consulting the operator is likewise a very rare exception. We have to date not observed signs of a possible gas embolism, for which Hong et al. demonstrated an incidence of 17% at the subclinical level (Hong et al. 2010).

Due to the position and the simultaneous capnoperitoneum, there is a risk of secondary tube displacement with subsequent unilateral

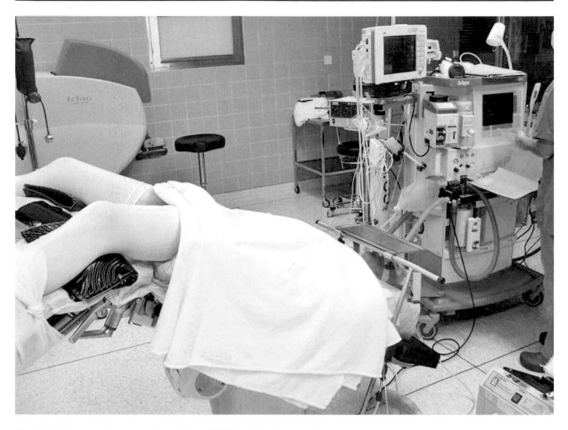

Fig. 2.4 The operation is performed in a 30° Trendelenburg position

ventilation. Therefore, accurate tube fixation is important. We have so far not observed laryngeal oedema necessitating immediate postoperative re-intubation and follow-up ventilation, as described by Phong et al. in a case report (Phong and Koh 2007).

An insufficient depth of anaesthesia constitutes a particular risk in this operation. Spontaneous movements of the patient during the operation could lead to substantial injuries as a result of the fixed settings of the ports. There is thus a need to ensure continuous control and monitoring of the depth of anaesthesia and relaxation. This can be achieved through individualised, patient-oriented, repeated administration of the opiate and the relaxant.

As part of the perioperative pain concept and to improve acceptance of the urinary catheter immediately after the operation, the patient is given intravenous metamizole [Novalgin®] 1 g and butylscopolamine [Buscopan®] 20 mg before terminating the anaesthesia. The infusions are opened after reversing the Trendelenburg positioning. Given stable haemodynamics, furosemide 20 mg i.v. is administered to achieve the urologically desirable flushing of the bladder.

2.3.4   Termination of Anaesthesia and Postoperative Monitoring

At the end of the operation, and given sufficient spontaneous breathing, the patient is extubated and moved to the recovery room for further monitoring by standard procedures for 1–2 h. Postoperative haemoglobin control by means of blood gas analysis is likewise standard. Fractionated doses of piritramide or clonidine are additionally administered in cases of catheter intolerance. The volume therapy is continued with an additional

1,000 ml crystalloid infusion [Sterofundin®]. The patient is returned to the ward as soon as his haemodynamics and vigilance allow.

2.3.5 Alternative Anaesthesia Management

To reduce postoperative drowsiness and thus improve patient comfort, intravenous anaesthesia with propofol and Ultiva is conceivable as an alternative anaesthetic procedure. On the one hand, however, dispensing with an inhalation anaesthetic necessitates valid neuromonitoring to avoid possible awareness, although this is more difficult owing to the position of the patient. On the other hand, continuous relaxation must be ensured in view of the risk of intraoperative injury in the event of spontaneous movements of the patient, meaning that intravenous relaxation by Perfusor and simultaneous relaxometric monitoring would be indispensable. In contrast, our experience shows that balanced general anaesthesia using a short-action inhalation anaesthetic, such as sevoflurane or desflurane, permits safe, easily controllable anaesthesia management requiring generally less monitoring. Nevertheless, attention should also be drawn to a study by Meininger et al., which shows that, under total intravenous anaesthesia management with corresponding monitoring and a fairly liberal infusion regime, creation of the capnoperitoneum and simultaneous Trendelenburg positioning does not result in any significant impairment of haemodynamics within a time frame of 4 h. One notable finding in this study is that no oedemas were seen to develop under the pre-induction volume therapy with crystalloid infusion at a rate of 10 ml/kg BW, followed by 6 ml/kg BW/h and the additional administration of colloidal infusion (Meininger et al. 2008).

Conclusion

The development of a standard for anaesthesia in robot-assisted prostatectomy permits good, safe perioperative patient care. Also important is comprehensive and, above all, timely information on possible cardiac risks of the patient, so that safe anaesthesia management can also be ensured in these cases. The task for the future will be to develop new approaches that make it possible to obtain information on the current state of cardiac health of the patient ahead of time, so that further cardiological diagnosis and therapy can, if necessary, be initiated without disrupting the existing operation schedule, thereby optimising the procedure and the safety of cardiac risk patients.

References

Falabella A, Moore-Jeffries E, Sullivan MJ, Nelson R, Lew M (2007) Cardiac function during steep Trendelenburg position and CO2 pneumoperitoneum for robotic-assisted prostatectomy: a trans-oesophageal Doppler probe study. Int J Med Robot 3(4):312–315

Hong JY, Kim WO, Kil HK (2010) Detection of subclinical CO(2) embolism by transesophageal echocardiography during laparoscopic radical prostatectomy. Urology 75(3):581–584, Epub 2009 Oct 30

Meininger D, Byhahn C (2008) Besonderheiten bei laparoskopischen Operationen aus anästhesiologischer Sicht. Anaesthesist 57:760–766. doi:10.1007/s00101-008-1422-y

Meininger D, Westphal K, Bremerich D, Runkel H, Probst M, Zwissler B, Byhahn C (2008) Effects of posture and prolonged pneumoperitoneum on hemodynamic parameters during laparoscopy. World J Surg 32:1400–1405. doi:10.1007/s00268-007-9424-5

Phong SV, Koh LK (2007) Anaesthesia for robotic-assisted radical prostatectomy: considerations for laparoscopy in the Trendelenburg position. Anaesth Intensive Care 35(2):281–285

Robotic Instruments

3

Jorn H. Witt and Mohan Nathan

EndoWrist® Instrumentation provides seven degrees of freedom for accomplishing precise tasks during robotic prostatectomy procedures with the *da Vinci*® Surgical System. The most frequently used EndoWrist® Instruments during Robotic-Assisted Radical Prostatectomy are listed below, along with several alternative instruments.

Frequently Used Instruments (Figs. 3.1, 3.2, 3.3, and 3.4):

Large Needle Driver (Fig. 3.1): for needle and suture manipulation. Many surgeons are using two needle drivers in both Robotic Instrument Arms. The use of only one needle driver and the needle manipulation with a dissector device (e.g. PK Dissecting Forceps or Maryland Bipolar Forceps) is not as comfortable but possible without real limitations in most situations.

Monopolar Curved Scissors (Fig. 3.2): allows additionally to the cutting function the use of monopolar energy.

PK Dissecting Forceps (Fig. 3.3): this instrument allows tissue manipulation and preparation as well as bipolar coagulation.

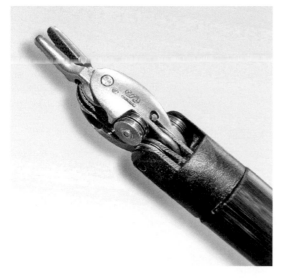

Fig. 3.1 Large Needle Drivers (2): used for suture ligation of dorsal vein complex and creation of urethrovesical anastomosis (held in both Left and Right Instrument Arms)

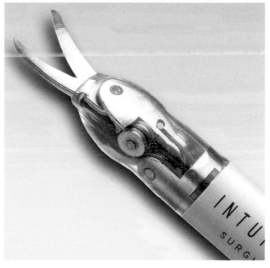

Fig. 3.2 *Hot Shears*™ (Monopolar Curved Scissors): used for cutting, dissecting, and monopolar coagulation (usually held in Right Instrument Arm)

H. John, et al. (eds.), *Atlas of Robotic Prostatectomy*,
DOI 10.1007/978-3-540-88408-8_3, © Springer-Verlag Berlin Heidelberg 2013

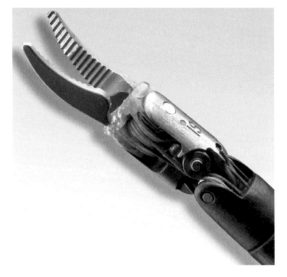

Fig. 3.3 *PK®* Dissecting Forceps: used for grasping, dissecting and bipolar coagulation (usually held in Left Instrument Arm)

ProGrasp™ (Fig. 3.4): allows grasping of tissue, applies traction e.g. to the prostate or can be used like a hook to retract e.g. the bladder. Is held in the 3rd Robotic Instrument Arm.

Alternative Robotic Instruments:

Maryland Bipolar Forceps – Fenestrated: alternative to *PK®* Dissector

Fenestrated Bipolar Forceps: alternative to Maryland Bipolar Forceps – Fenestrated

Round Tip Scissors: alternative to *HotShears*™ for dissecting and cutting

Permanent Cautery Hook: alternative to *HotShears*™ for dissecting and coagulation

SutureCut™ Needle Driver: alternative to Large Needle Driver

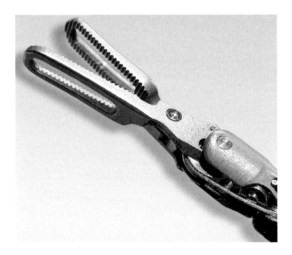

Fig. 3.4 *ProGrasp*™: holding and traction device, used in the 3rd Robotic Instrument Arm

Surgical Steps

4

Hubert John, Peter Wiklund, and Jorn H. Witt

with contributions from Thomas E. Ahlering, Randy Fagin, Rolf Gillitzer, Mani Menon, Alexander Mottrie, Vipul R. Patel, Bernardo Rocco, Charles-Henry Rochat, Alok Shrivastava, Stefan Siemer, Michael Stöckle, Gerald Tan, Ashutosh K. Tewari, Joachim W. Thüroff, Christian Wagner, and Vahudin Zugor

4.1 Port Placement

4.1.1 Extraperitoneal

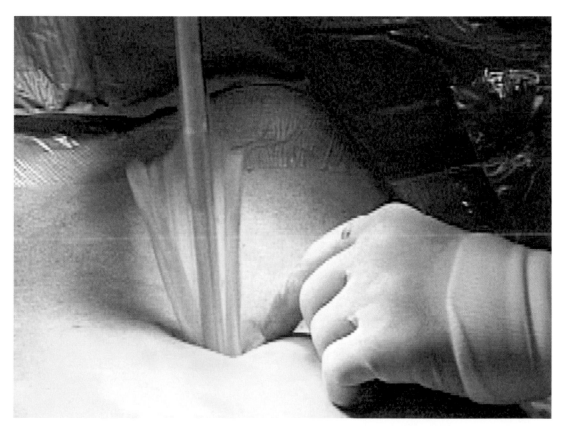

Fig. 4.1 Balloon dilatation of the extraperitoneal space

H. John, et al. (eds.), *Atlas of Robotic Prostatectomy*,
DOI 10.1007/978-3-540-88408-8_4, © Springer-Verlag Berlin Heidelberg 2013

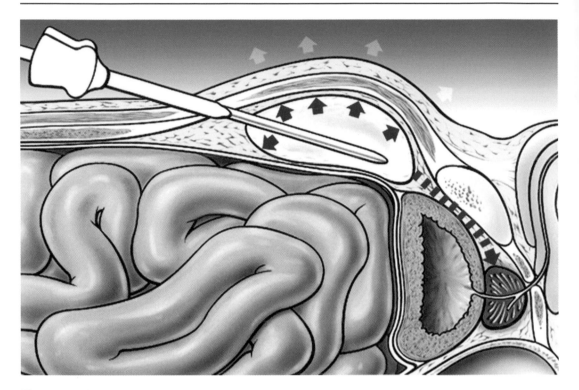

Fig. 4.1 (continued)

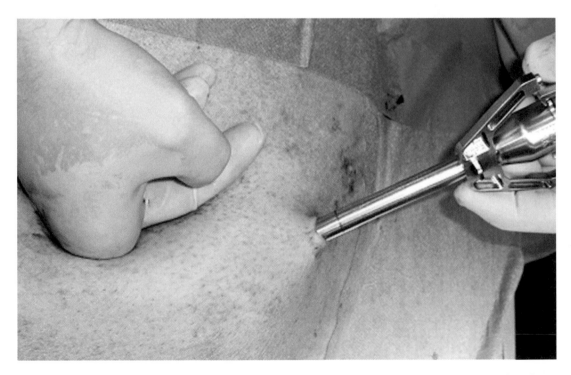

Fig. 4.2 First robotic trocar placement. The tip of the right index finger guides the blunt obturator tip of the 8 mm trocar down into the extraperitoneal space, which has been created by prior balloon dilatation

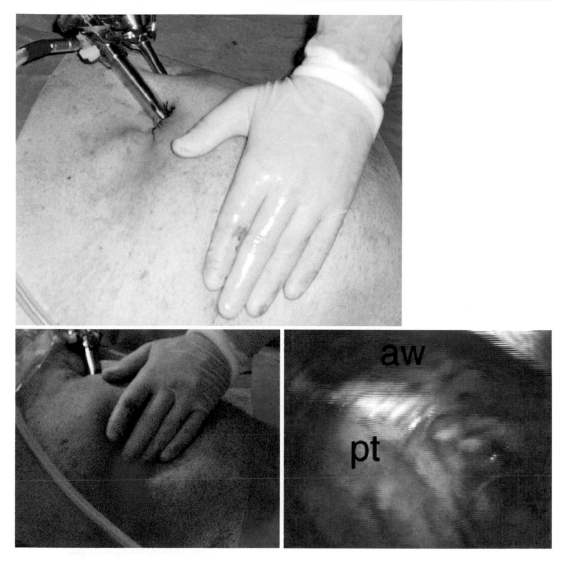

Fig. 4.3   Expanding the extraperitoneal space

4.1.2 Transperitoneal

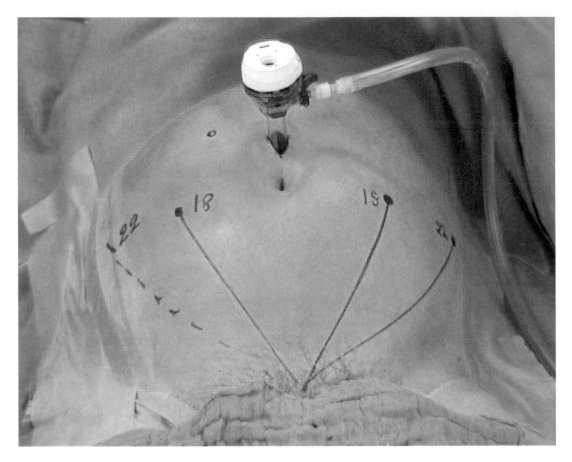

Fig. 4.4 Supraumbilical access and positioning of the ports

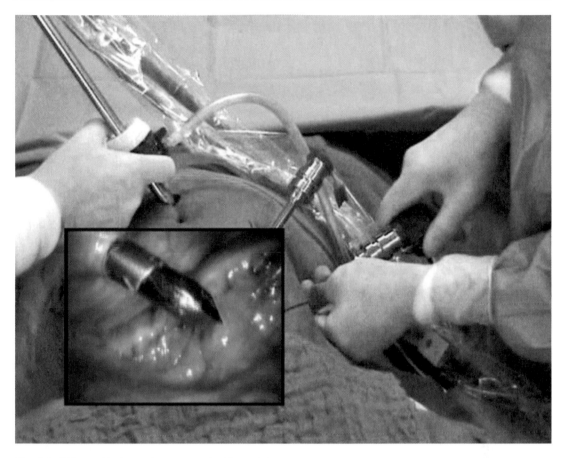

Fig. 4.5   Video-guided port placement under direct vision

4.2 Cavum Retzii

4.2.1 Normal

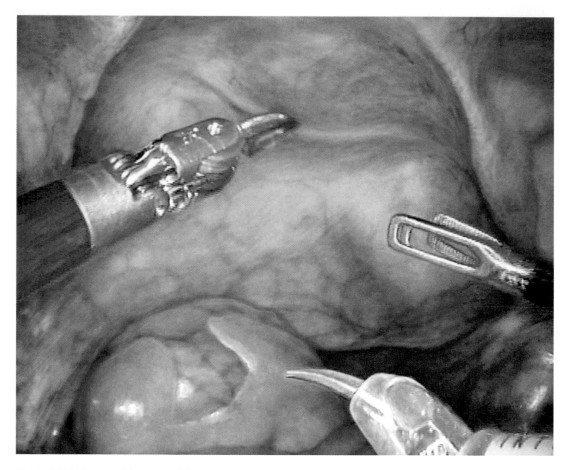

Fig. 4.6 Initial view of the space of Douglas. The entrance to the cavum retzii is still closed

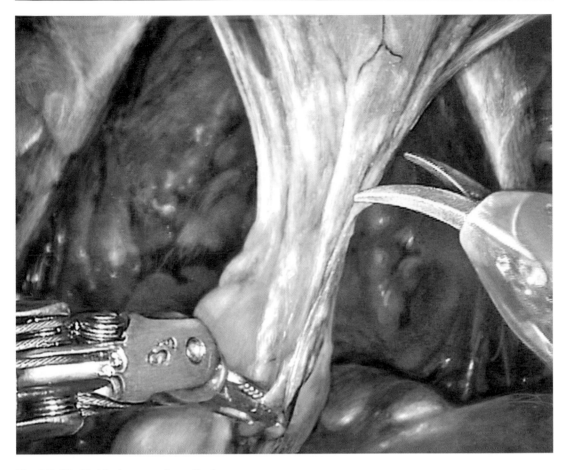

Fig. 4.7 The bladder is extraperitonealised

4.2.2 Special

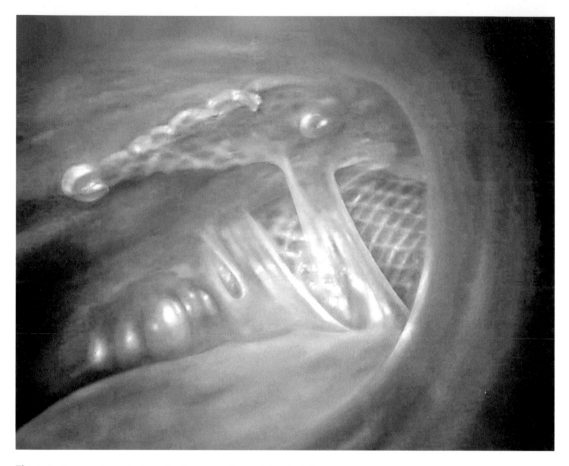

Fig. 4.8 Transperitoneal view after laparoscopic mesh implantation

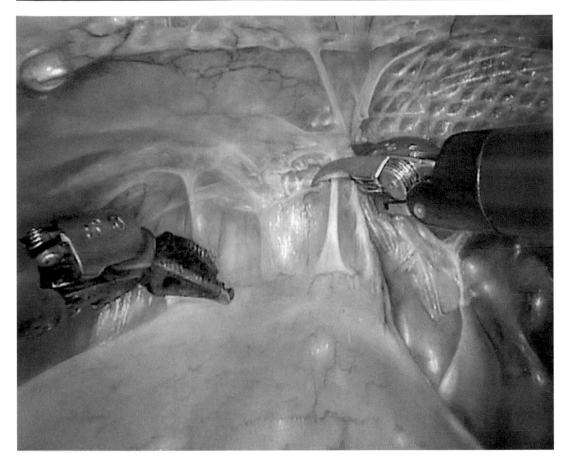

Fig. 4.9 Adhesiolysis of fibrotic adhesions between the implanted mesh and small intestine

4.3   Lymphadenectomy

4.3.1   Limited Lymphadenectomy

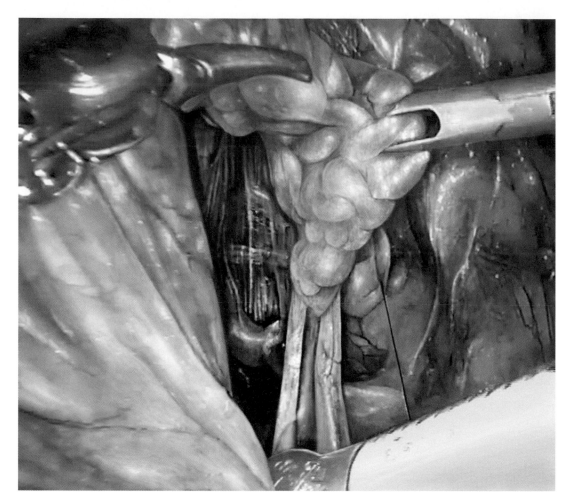

Fig. 4.10 Lymph nodes between the iliac vein and the fossa obturatoria

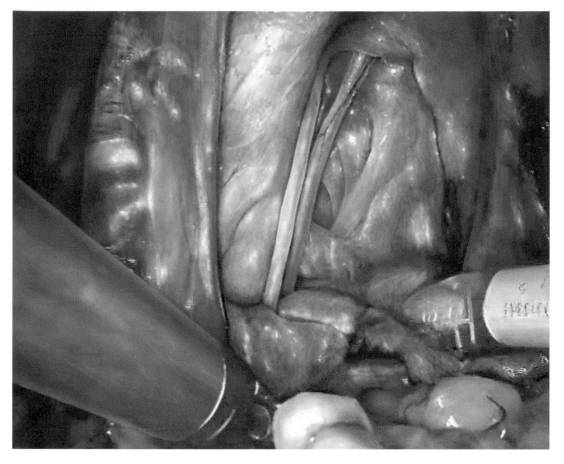

Fig. 4.11 Fossa obturatoria following limited lymph node dissection

4.3.2 Extended Lymphadenectomy

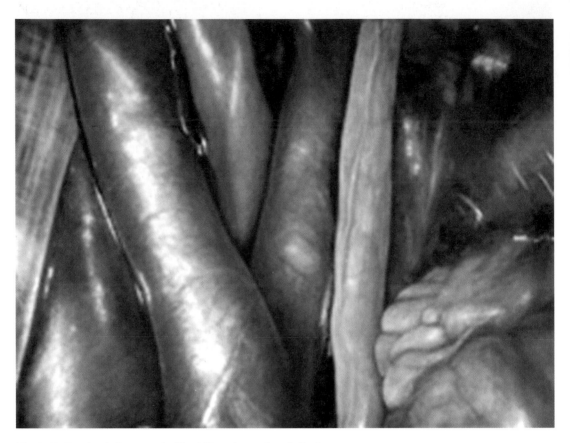

Fig. 4.12 Proximal view onto the iliac bifurcation and medialised ureter

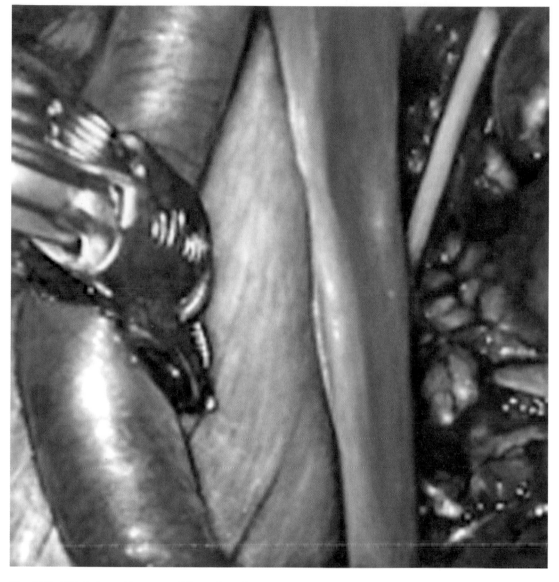

Fig. 4.13 Distal view with separated iliac vein and artery

4.4 Endopelvic Fascia

4.4.1 Incision

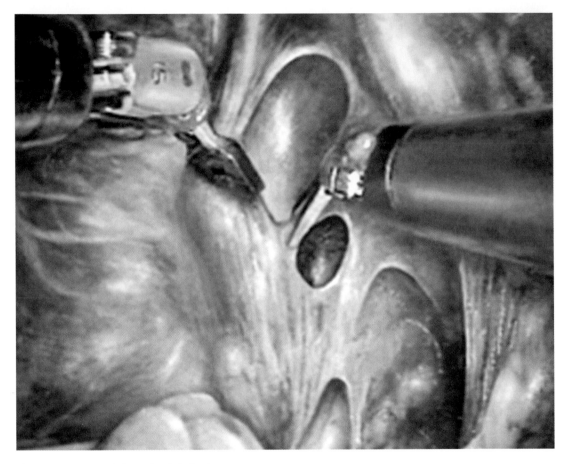

Fig. 4.14 Incision of the endopelvic fascia

4.4.2   Accessory Pudendal Vessels

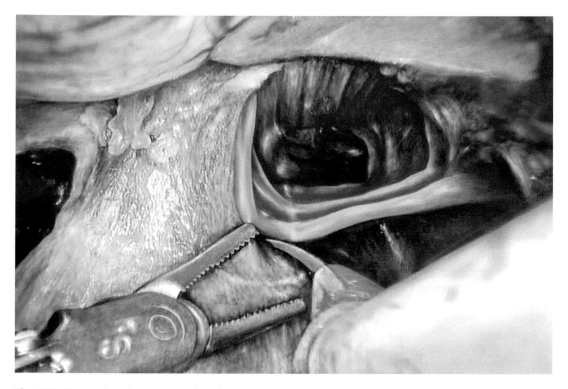

Fig. 4.15 Preparetion of accessory pudendal vessels

4.5   Dorsal Vascular Complex

4.5.1   Exposition and Incision

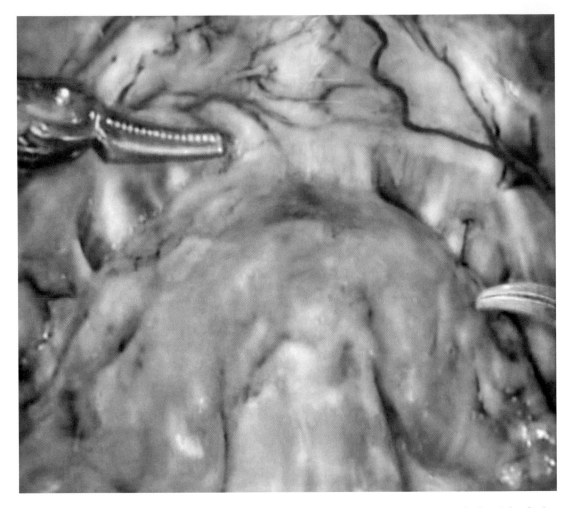

Fig. 4.16 The trigone between both endopelvic fascias and the dorsal venous complex is de-fatted for further dissection

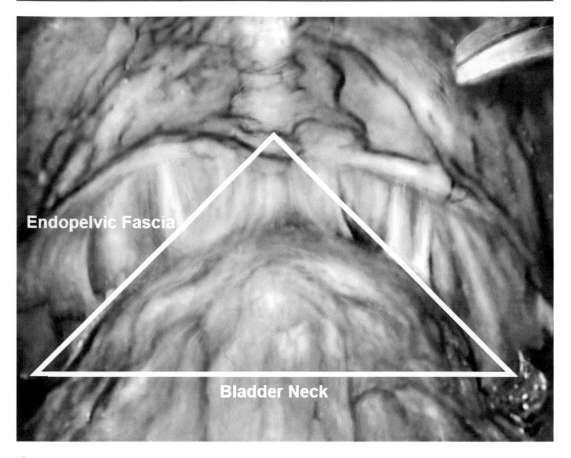

Fig. 4.16   (continued)

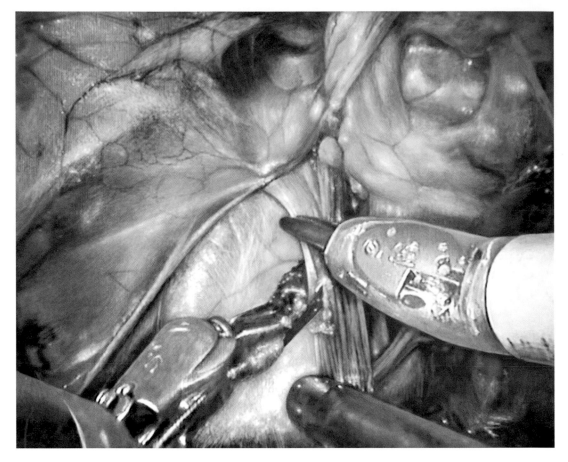

Fig. 4.17 Incision of the endopelvic fascia and exposure of the dorsal vascular complex

4.5.2   Ligature and Stapler

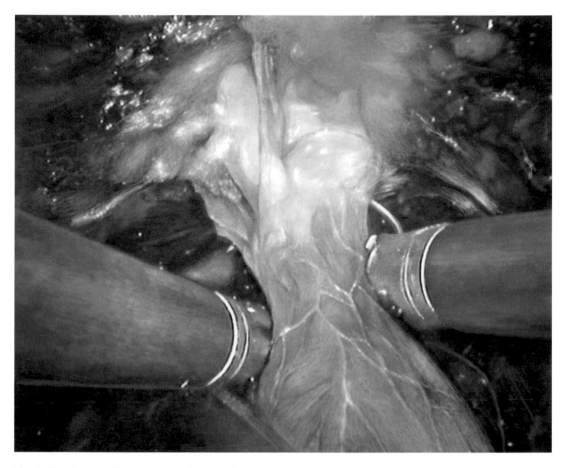

Fig. 4.18   Ligation of the dorsal vascular complex

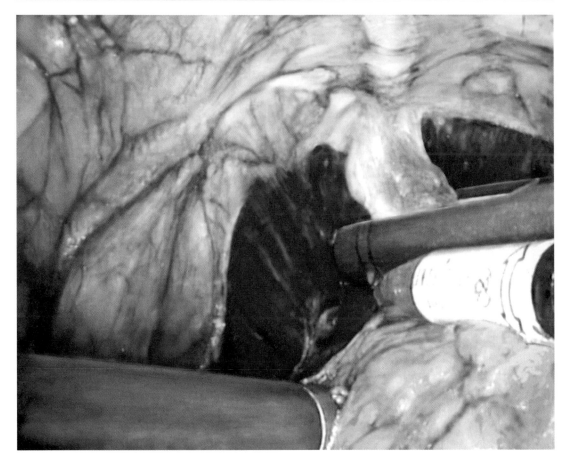

Fig. 4.19 Stapling of the dorsal vascular complex

4.6 Pubovesical Ligaments

4.6.1 Pubovesical Ligaments: Incision

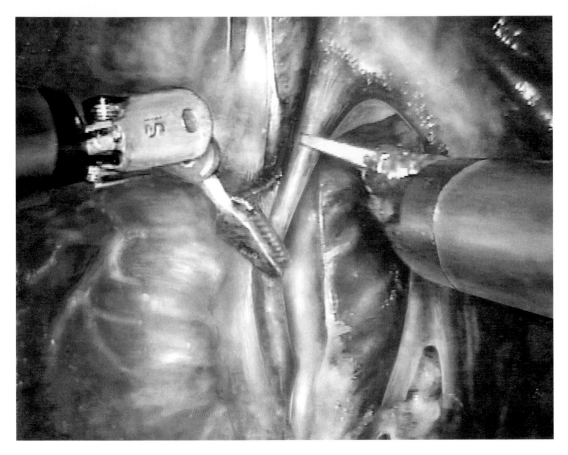

Fig. 4.20 Incision of the right pubovesical ligament

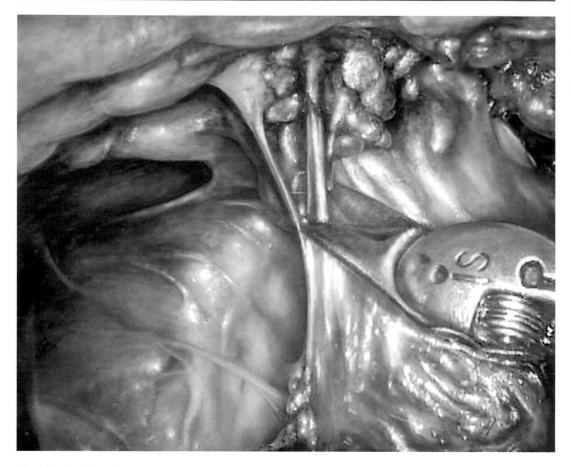

Fig. 4.21 Incision of the left pubovesical ligaments

4.7 Bladder Neck Dissection

4.7.1 Normal Situs

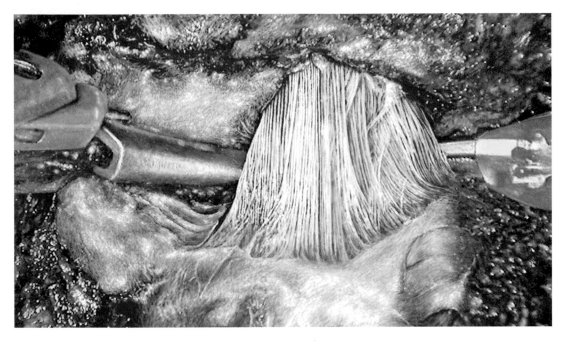

Fig. 4.22 Proximal urethra, normal

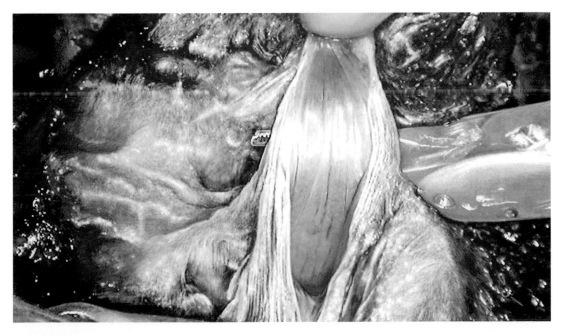

Fig. 4.23 Proximal urethra normal, "scissor-blade sign"

4.7.2   Large Gland

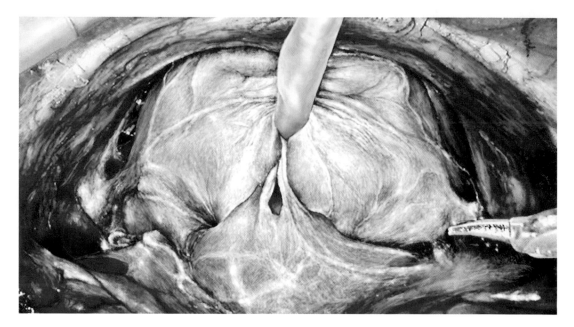

Fig. 4.24   Bladder neck of a large prostate

4.7.3   Median Lobe

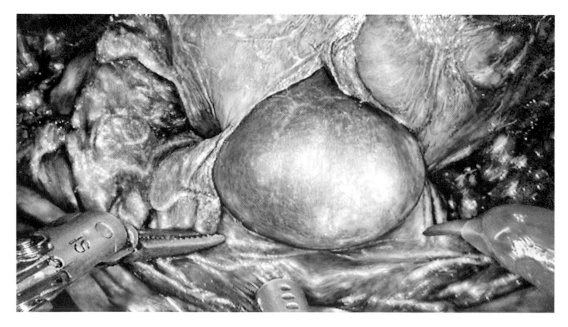

Fig. 4.25   Presentation of a large median lobe after bladder neck opening

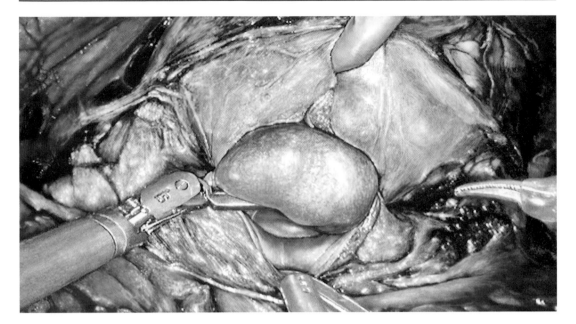

Fig. 4.26 Exposure of the median lobe

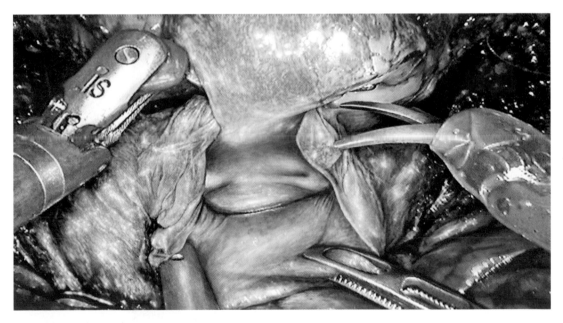

Fig. 4.27 Complete dissection of the median lobe from the bladder neck

4.8   Vas Deferens, Seminal Vesicles

4.8.1   Vesico-Prostatic Muscle

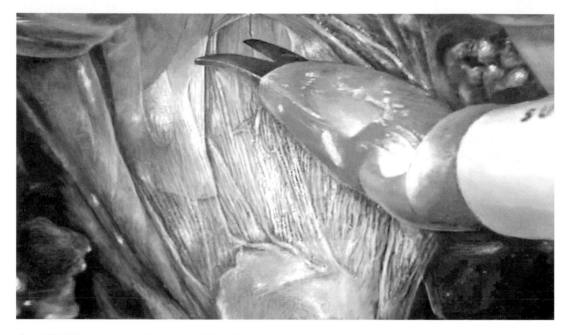

Fig. 4.28 The vesico-prostatic muscle is incised

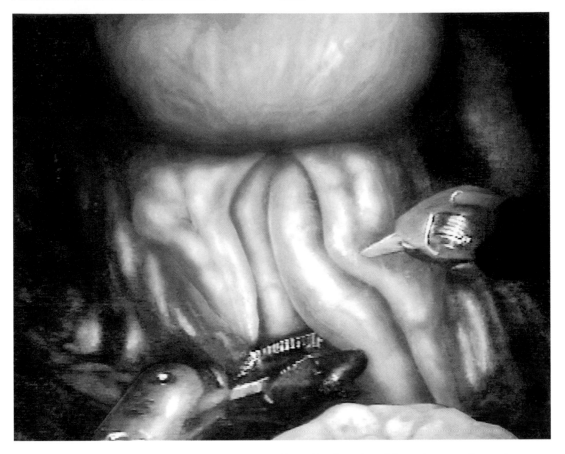

Fig. 4.29 Exposure of the vasa deferentia and seminal vesicles after dissection of the vesico-prostatic muscle

4.8.2 Partial Seminal Vesical Sparing Technique

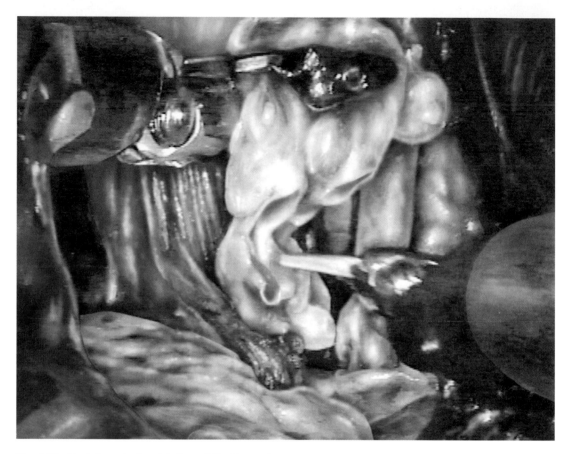

Fig. 4.30 The left seminal vesicle is partially dissected

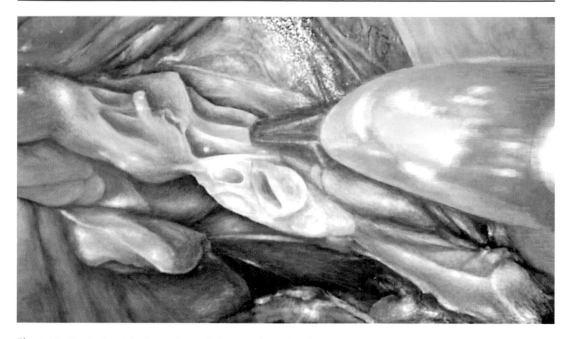

Fig. 4.31 Seminal vesicle tip-sparing technique on the *right side*

4.9 Retroprostatic Dissection

4.9.1 Posterior Prostatic Fascia (Denonvilliers)

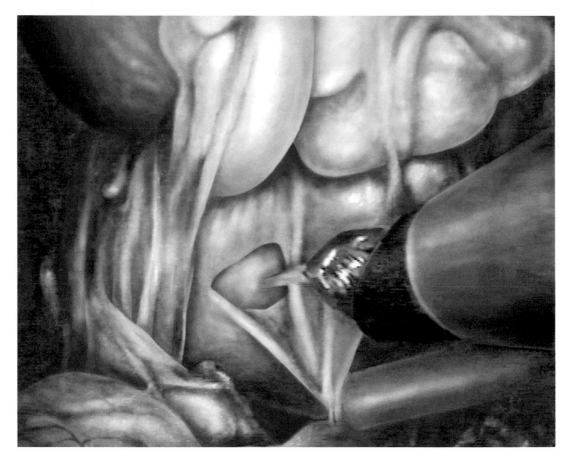

Fig. 4.32 Incision of the posterior prostatic fascia

4.9.2   Dorsal Development to the Apex

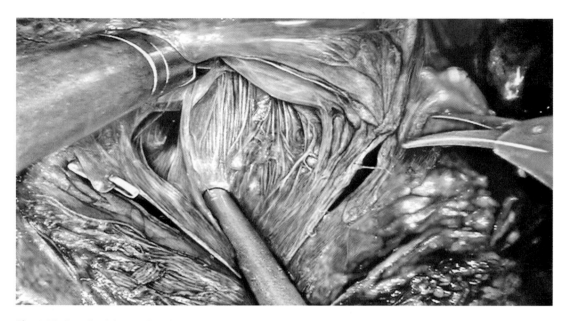

Fig. 4.33 Intrafascial posterior dissection between the prostatic capsule and the posterior prostatic fascia

4.10   Neurovascular Bundle

4.10.1   Prostatic pedicles

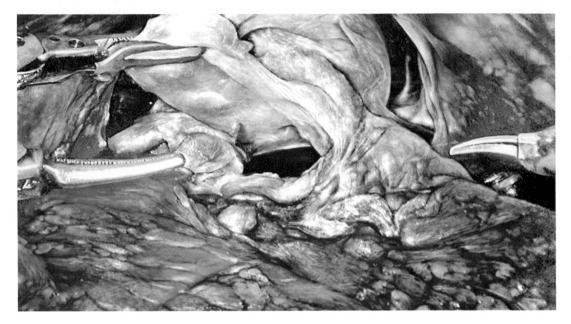

Fig. 4.34 Exposure of the right prostatic pedicle

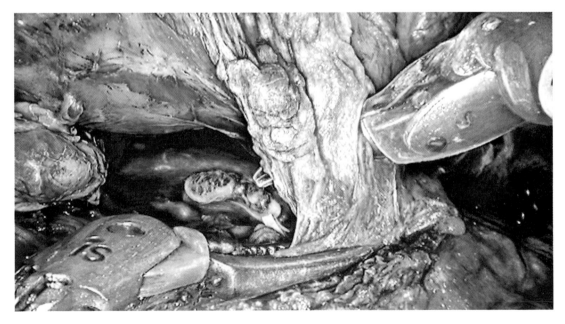

Fig. 4.35 Preparation of the prostatic pedicle on the *right side*

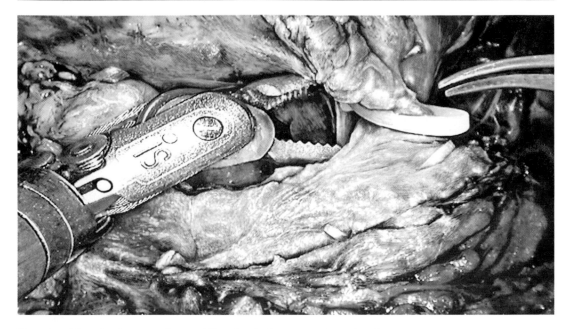

Fig. 4.36 Dissection between clips, avoiding electrical energy, on the *right side*

4.10.2   Retrograde Technique

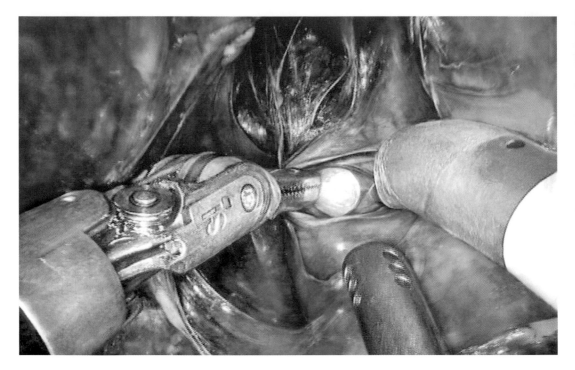

Fig. 4.37 The neurovascular bundle is released apically

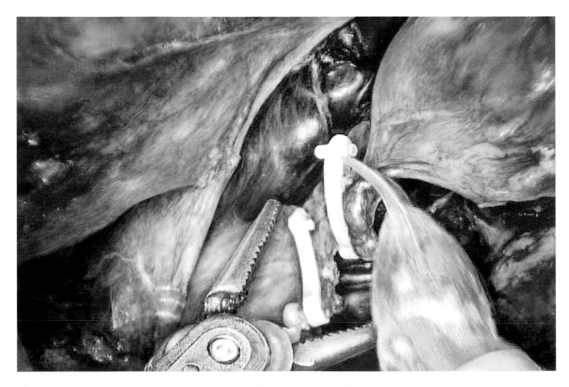

Fig. 4.38 After retrograde release of the neurovascular structures the left pedicle is divided

4.10.3 Antegrade Technique

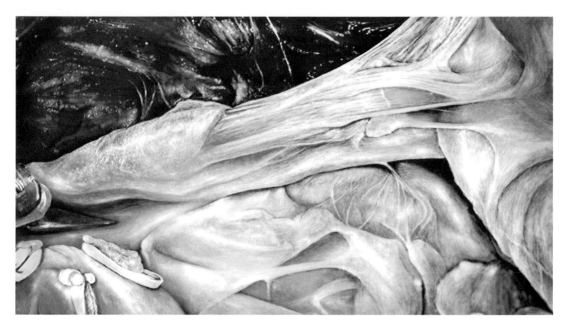

Fig. 4.39 Left intrafascial descending dissection

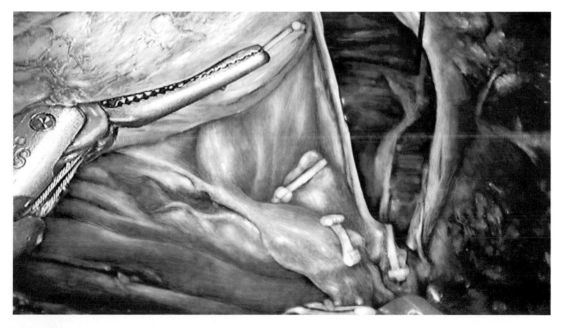

Fig. 4.40 Antegrade nerve sparing on the *right side*

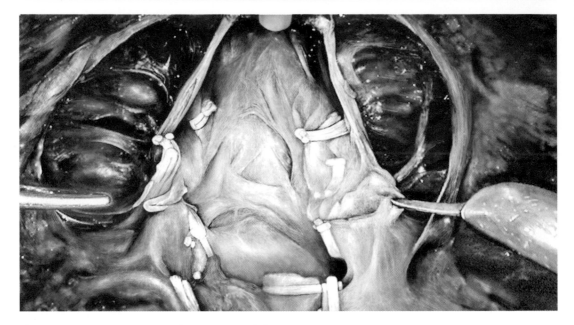

Fig. 4.41 The neurovascular bundles are preserved bilaterally

4.11 Apical Dissection

4.11.1 Ventral Aspect

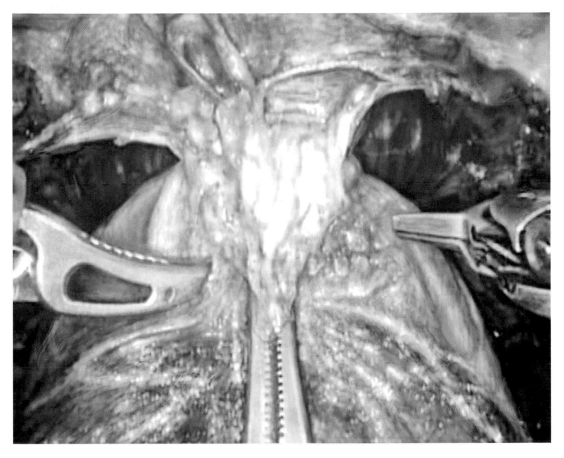

Fig. 4.42 The urethra is exposed by slight tension of the specimen

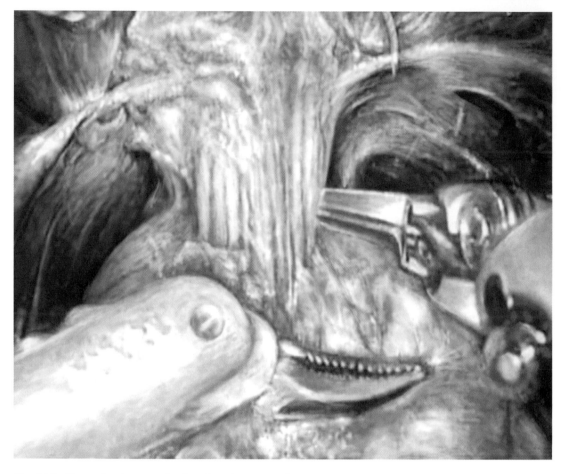

Fig. 4.43 The urethra is exposed and ready to be transected

4.11.2   Dorsal Aspect

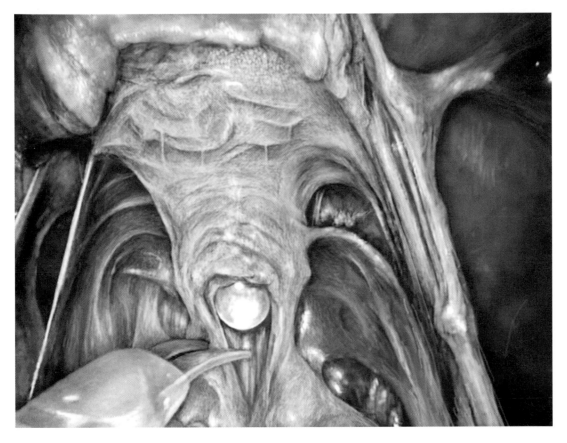

Fig. 4.44   The dorsal urethra is transected

4.12   Anastomotic Techniques

4.12.1   Single Knot Suturing

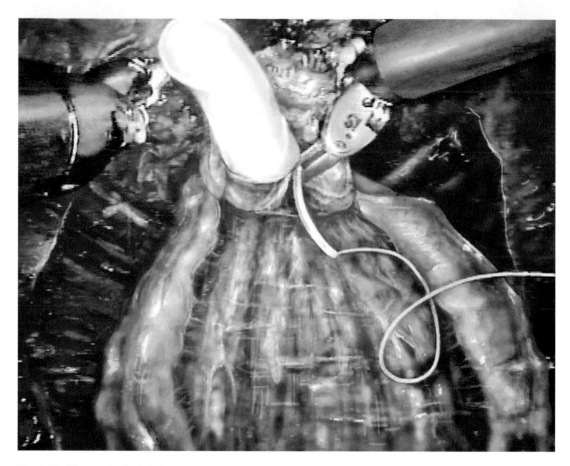

Fig. 4.45 First urethral stitch, inside-out

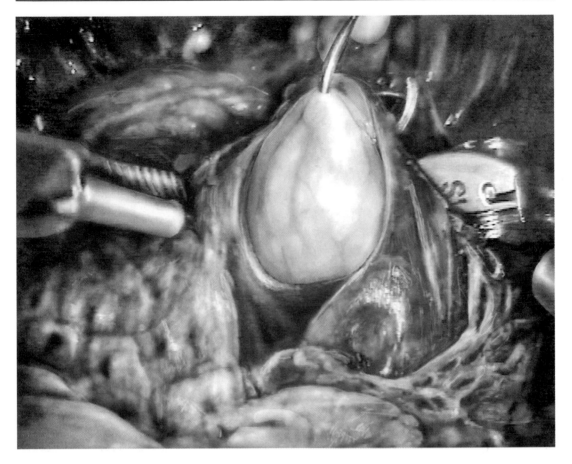

Fig. 4.46 First bladder stitch, outside-in

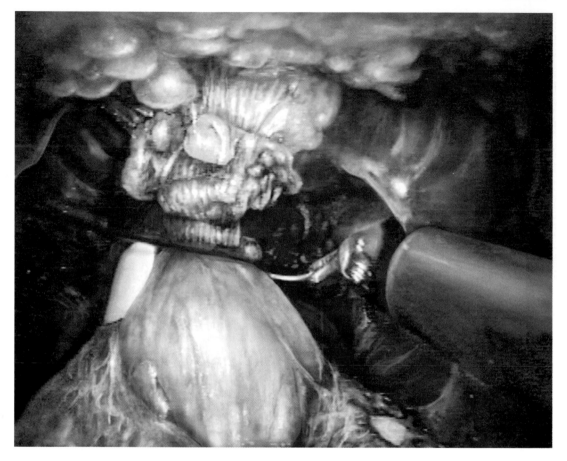

Fig. 4.47 The dorsal anastomotic plate is sutured

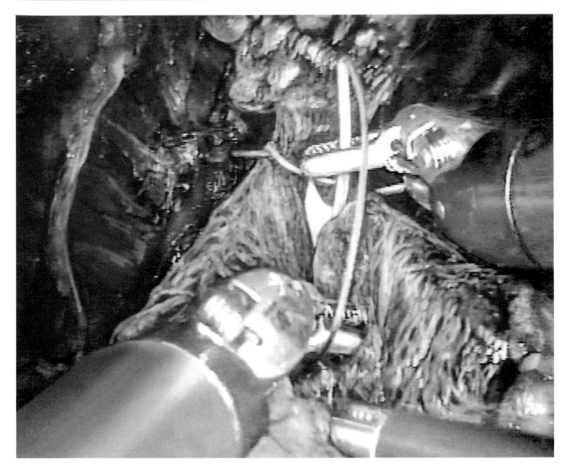

Fig. 4.48 Final ventral stitch

4.12.2   Running Suture

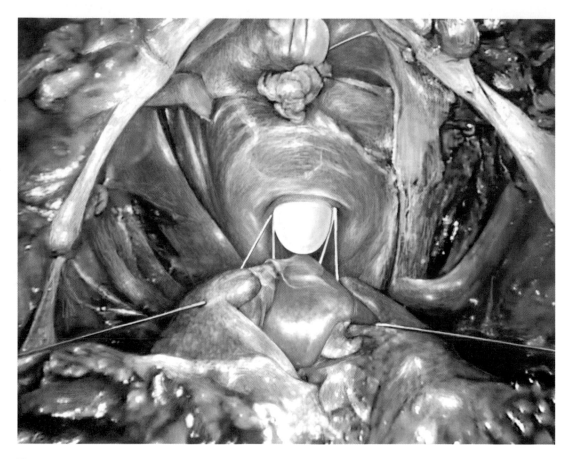

Fig. 4.49 Single layer continuous anastomosis, before the bladder neck is drawn down to the urethral stump

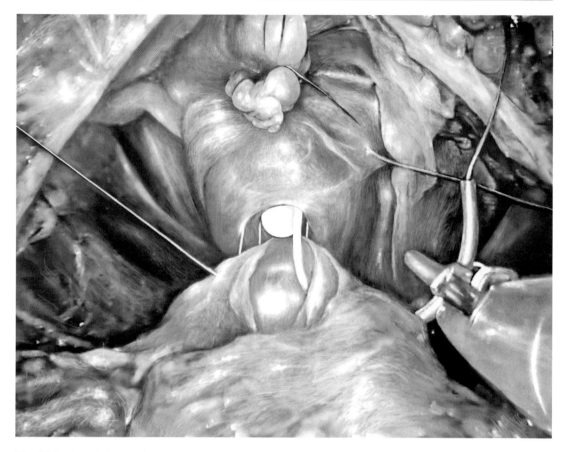

Fig. 4.50 Ventral closure after approximation of the dorsal plate

4.13 Additional Concepts for Functional Restoration

4.13.1 Dorsal Reconstruction

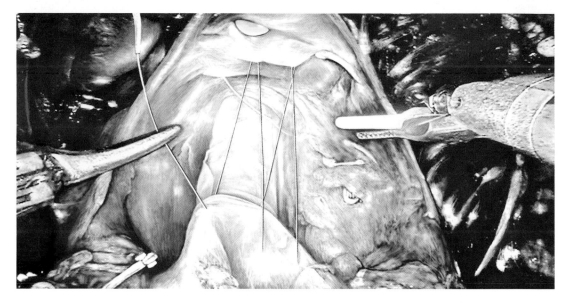

Fig. 4.51 The sutures are laid between the prostatic fascia of the dorsal urethra and the bladder neck

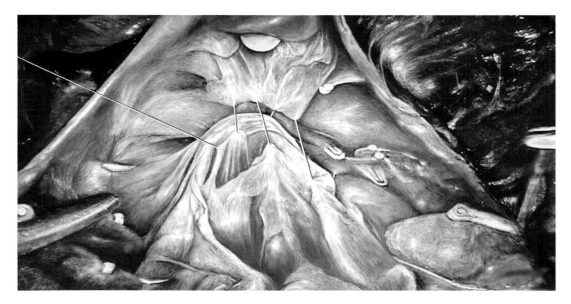

Fig. 4.52 Adaption of the resected posterior prostatic fascia

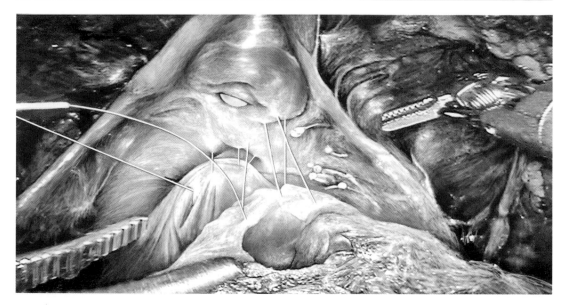

Fig. 4.53 Double layer dorsal reconstruction

4.13.2 Ventral Suspension

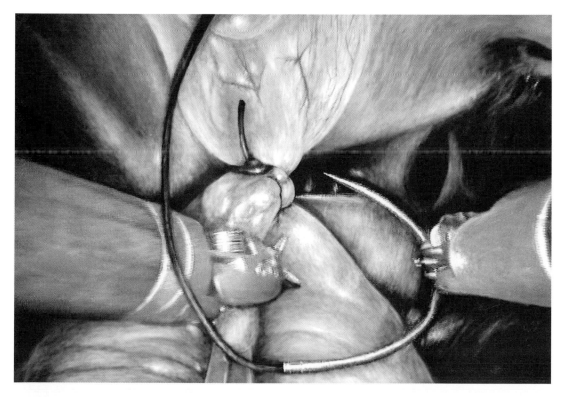

Fig. 4.54 Beginning at the puboprostatic ligament

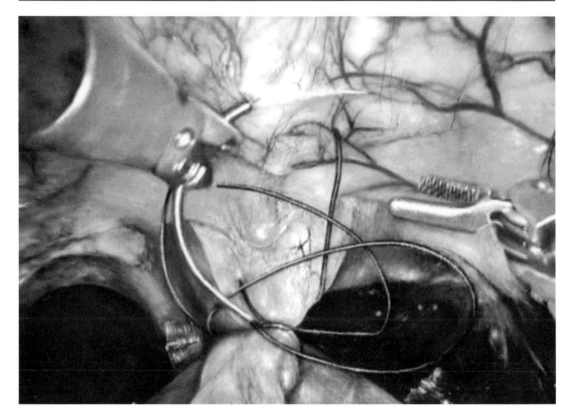

Fig. 4.55 Stitch through the periosteum of the symphysis

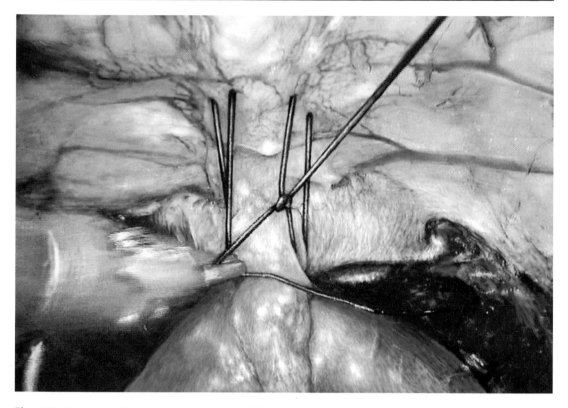

Fig. 4.56   Gentle elevation at the urethra using a sliding knot

4.13.3 Ventral Reconstruction

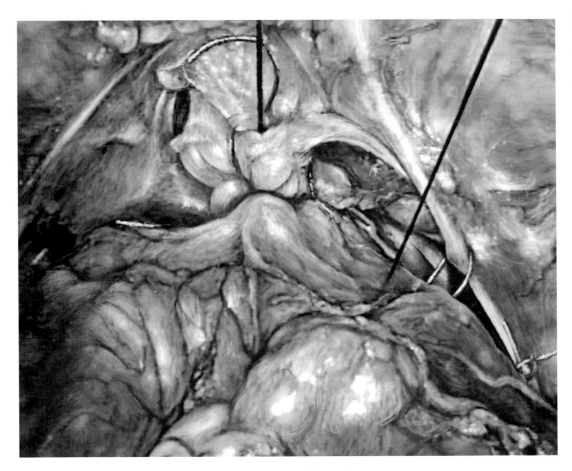

Fig. 4.57 Adaption of the lateral bladder aspect to the endopelvic fascia

4.14 Complications

4.14.1 Rectal Lesion

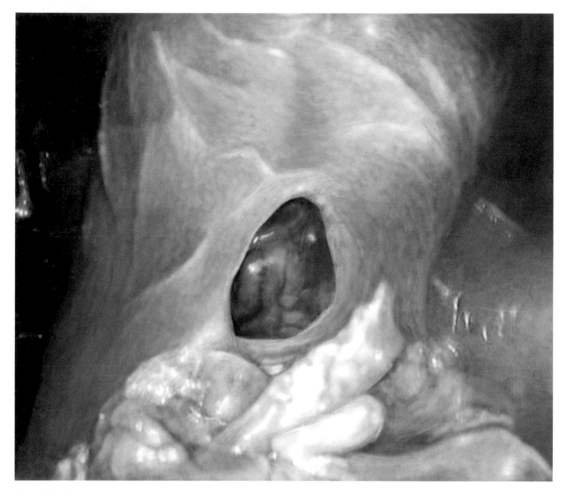

Fig. 4.58 Rectal lesion

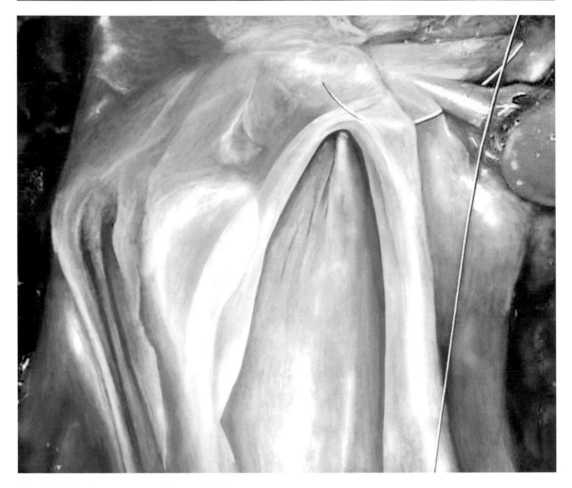

Fig. 4.59 Continuous suture of the rectal lesion

4.14.2   Iliac Vein Lesion

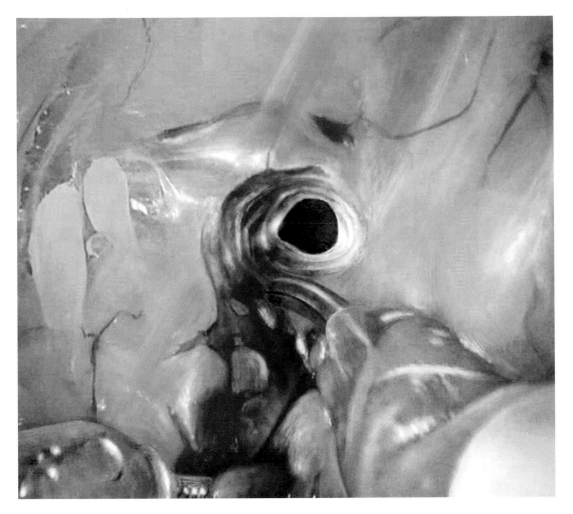

Fig. 4.60 Iliac vein lesion

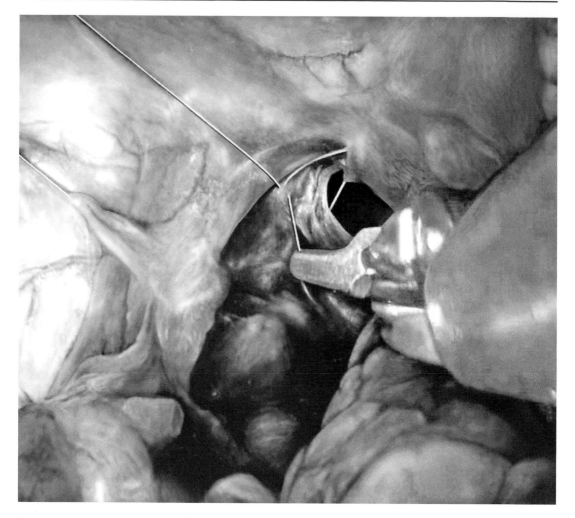

Fig. 4.61 Continuous suture of the iliac vein lesion

Index

H. John, et al. (eds.), *Atlas of Robotic Prostatectomy*,
DOI 10.1007/978-3-540-88408-8, © Springer-Verlag Berlin Heidelberg 2013

Printing and Binding: Stürtz GmbH, Würzburg